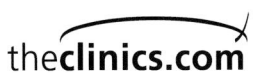
theclinics.com

VETERINARY CLINICS

OF NORTH AMERICA

Small Animal Practice

Effective Communication
in Veterinary Practice

GUEST EDITORS
Karen K. Cornell, DVM, PhD
Jennifer C. Brandt, MSW, LISW, PhD
Kathleen A. Bonvicini, MPH

January 2007 • Volume 37 • Number 1

SAUNDERS

An Imprint of Elsevier, Inc.
PHILADELPHIA   LONDON   TORONTO   MONTREAL   SYDNEY   TOKYO

W.B. SAUNDERS COMPANY
A Division of Elsevier Inc.

Elsevier, Inc., 1600 John F. Kennedy Blvd., Suite 1800, Philadelphia, PA 19103-2899

http://www.vetsmall.theclinics.com

VETERINARY CLINICS OF NORTH AMERICA:	**Volume 37, Number 1**
SMALL ANIMAL PRACTICE	**ISSN 0195-5616**
January 2007	**ISBN-13: 978-1-4160-4382-9**
Editor: John Vassallo; j.vassallo@elsevier.com	**ISBN-10: 1-4160-4382-9**

The ideas and opinions expressed in *Veterinary Clinics of North America: Small Animal Practice* do not necessarily reflect those of the Publisher. The Publisher does not assume any responsibility for any injury and/or damage to persons or property arising out of or related to any use of the material contained in this periodical. The reader is advised to check the appropriate medical literature and the product information currently provided by the manufacturer of each drug to be administered to verify the dosage, the method and duration of administration, or contraindications. It is the responsibility of the treating physician or other health care professional, relying on independent experience and knowledge of the patient, to determine drug dosages and the best treatment for the patient. Mention of any product in this issue should not be construed as endorsement by the contributors, editors, or the Publisher of the product or manufacturers' claims.

Veterinary Clinics of North America: Small Animal Practice (ISSN 0195-5616) is published bimonthly (For Post Office use only: volume 36 issue 5 of 6) by Elsevier Inc., 360 Park Avenue South, New York, NY 10010-1710. Months of issue are January, March, May, July, September, and November. Business and Editorial offices: 1600 John F. Kennedy Blvd., Suite 1800, Philadelphia, PA 19103-2899. Customer Service Office: 6277 Sea Harbor Drive, Orlando, FL 32887-4800. Periodicals postage paid at New York, NY and additional mailing offices. Subscription prices are $187.00 per year for US individuals, $297.00 per year for US institutions, $94.00 per year for US students and residents, $248.00 per year for Canadian individuals, $373.00 per year for Canadian institutions, $259.00 per year for international individuals, $373.00 per year for international institutions and $127.00 per year for Canadian and foreign students/residents. To receive student/resident rate, orders must be accompanied by name of affiliated institution, date of term, and the *signature* of program/residency coordinator on institution letterhead. Orders will be billed at individual rate until proof of status is received. Foreign air speed delivery is included in all *Clinics* subscription prices. All prices are subject to change without notice. **POSTMASTER**: Send address changes to *Veterinary Clinics of North America: Small Animal Practice*, Elsevier Periodicals Customer Service, 6277 Sea Harbor Drive, Orlando, FL 32887-4800, USA; phone: 1-800-654-2452 [toll free number for US customers], or (+1)(407) 345-4000 [customers outside US]; fax: (+1)(407) 363-1354; email: usjcs@elsevier.com.

Veterinary Clinics of North America: Small Animal Practice is also published in Japanese by Inter Zoo Publishing Co., Ltd., Aoyama Crystal-Bldg 5F, 3-5-12 Kitaaoyama, Minato-ku, Tokyo 107-0061, Japan.

Reprints: For copies of 100 or more, of articles in this publication, please contact the Commercial Reprints Department, Elsevier Inc., 360 Park Avenue South, New York, New York 10010-1710. Tel. (212) 633-3813 Fax: (212) 462-1935, email: reprints@elsevier.com

Veterinary Clinics of North America: Small Animal Practice is covered in *Current Contents/Agriculture, Biology and Environmental Sciences, Science Citation Index, ASCA, Index Medicus, Excerpta Medica,* and *BIOSIS.*

Printed in the United States of America.

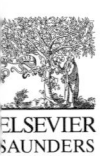
ELSEVIER
SAUNDERS

VETERINARY CLINICS
SMALL ANIMAL PRACTICE

Effective Communication in Veterinary Practice

GUEST EDITORS

KAREN K. CORNELL, DVM, PhD, Diplomate, American College of Veterinary Surgeons; Department of Small Animal Medicine and Surgery, College of Veterinary Medicine, University of Georgia, Athens, Georgia

JENNIFER C. BRANDT, MSW, LISW, PhD, Program Director, Honoring the Bond, and Adjunct Associate Professor, Veterinary Clinical Sciences, College of Veterinary Medicine, The Ohio State University, Columbus, Ohio

KATHLEEN A. BONVICINI, MPH, Associate Director of Education and Research, Institute for Healthcare Communication, New Haven, Connecticut

CONTRIBUTORS

SARAH K. ABOOD, DVM, PhD, Coordinator, Student Programs, and Assistant Professor, Small Animal Clinical Sciences, College of Veterinary Medicine, Michigan State University, East Lansing, Michigan

CINDY L. ADAMS, MSW, PhD, Associate Professor of Veterinary Medicine-Clinical Communication, Faculty of Veterinary Medicine, University of Calgary, Calgary, Alberta, Canada

SHANE W. BATEMAN, DVM, DVSc, Diplomate, American College of Veterinary Emergency and Critical Care; Clinical Associate Professor and Head, Small Animal Care and Wellness Section, Department of Veterinary Clinical Sciences, The Ohio State University, Columbus, Ohio

KATHLEEN A. BONVICINI, MPH, Associate Director of Education and Research, Institute for Healthcare Communication, New Haven, Connecticut

JENNIFER C. BRANDT, MSW, LISW, PhD, Program Director, Honoring the Bond, and Adjunct Associate Professor, Veterinary Clinical Sciences, College of Veterinary Medicine, The Ohio State University, Columbus, Ohio

CECILE A. CARSON, MD, Clinical Associate Professor of Medicine and Psychiatry, University of Rochester Medical Center, Honeyoe, New York

SUSAN P. COHEN, DSW, Director of Counseling, The Animal Medical Center, New York, New York

KAREN K. CORNELL, DVM, PhD, Diplomate, American College
of Veterinary Surgeons; Department of Small Animal Medicine and
Surgery, College of Veterinary Medicine, University of Georgia, Athens,
Georgia

RICHARD M. DeBOWES, DVM, MS, Diplomate, American College of Veterinary
Surgeons; Professor of Surgery, and Associate Dean, External Relations and
Development, Veterinary Clinical Sciences, College of Veterinary Medicine,
Washington State University, Pullman, Washington

RICHARD M. FRANKEL, PhD, Professor of Medicine and Geriatrics, and Senior
Research Scientist, Regenstrief Institute, Indiana University School of Medicine,
Indianapolis, Indiana

CHANDRA M. GRABILL, PhD, Licensed Psychologist, Office of Academic Programs
and Student Services, Michigan State University College of Veterinary Medicine,
East Lansing, Michigan

MICHELLE KOPCHA, DVM, MS, Associate Professor, Department of Large Animal
Clinical Sciences, Practice Based Ambulatory Program, Michigan State University,
East Lansing, Michigan

DONALD J. KLINGBORG, DVM, Associate Dean for Extension and Public
Programs, and Director, Center for Continuing Professional Education,
School of Veterinary Medicine, University of California at Davis, Davis,
California

JON KLINGBORG, DVM, Valley Veterinary Clinic, Merced, California

LAUREL LAGONI, MS, President/CEO, World by the Tail, Inc., and Director,
www.PetPeopleHelp.com, Fort Collins, Colorado

MICHAEL McDONALD, PhD, Professor and Maurice Young Chair of Applied Ethics,
The W. Maurice Young Centre for Applied Ethics, The University of British
Columbia, Vancouver, British Columbia, Canada

CAROL A. MORGAN, DVM, Doctoral Candidate, Interdisciplinary Studies Graduate
Program, The University of British Columbia, Vancouver, British Columbia,
Canada

JAMES K. MORRISEY, DVM, Diplomate–Avian Practice; American Board of
Veterinary Practitioners Lecturer, Section of Wildlife and Exotic Medicine,
Department of Clinical Sciences, College of Veterinary Medicine,
Cornell University, Ithaca, New York

DANIEL O'CONNELL, PhD, Regional Consultant, Institute for Healthcare
Communication, New Haven, Connecticut; Principal, Training, Coaching and
Consultation Group; Clinical Instructor, University of Washington School of
Medicine, Seattle, Washington

KATHLEEN L. RUBY, MEd, PhD, Assistant Professor and Director, Department of Counseling, Wellness and Leadership, College of Veterinary Medicine, Washington State University, Pullman, Washington

JANE R. SHAW, DVM, PhD, Director, Argus Institute, and Assistant Professor of Veterinary Communication, James L. Voss Veterinary Teaching Hospital, Colorado State University, Fort Collins, Colorado

BONITA VOILAND, MS, MBA, Assistant Dean of Hospital Operations, Cornell University Hospital for Animals, Ithaca, New York

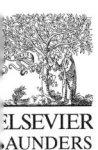

VETERINARY CLINICS
SMALL ANIMAL PRACTICE

Effective Communication in Veterinary Practice

CONTENTS VOLUME 37 • NUMBER 1 • JANUARY 2007

> Effective communication is necessary for achieving important outcomes in veterinary practice, including patient health, accuracy, efficiency, and economic viability. Communication is a series of learned skills. Daily practice, feedback, and refinement are the ingredients for continued practice success.

> Effective veterinary health care teams are crucial to the successful practice of veterinary medicine and contribute greatly to everything from excellent patient and client care to practice financial stability and practitioner and staff quality of work life. Contrary to a commonly held belief, healthy teams do not form naturally. This article examines the complex nature of successful teams and outlines a process that can be followed to assist practices in their efforts to evolve from ordinary work groups to highly interactive teams.

> This article reviews three decision-making models for veterinary–client and physician–patient interactions and proposes adaptation of the 4E communication model from human medicine for application in veterinary–client interactions. These models incorporate specific communication skills for achieving the four components of a client interview: engagement, empathy, education, and enlistment.

Treating nonverbal communication with the thoughtfulness and observation with which we approach any other clinical problem can produce a set of skills that can be applied in every encounter. Skill development begins first with enhancing one's observations of nonverbal behavior and then diagnosing whether or not the client is feeling safe. Using one or more of the nonverbal skills when clients are feeling not-safe creates more satisfaction for the client and veterinarian and motivates clients to become full partners in their animal's care.

As veterinarians, effective interactions with clients and coworkers are fundamental to our professional satisfaction and success. This article first reviews the basis of a difficult interaction and provides specific communication skills to help the veterinarian more successfully manage situations that he or she may find difficult. Then, the authors offer exercises to assist veterinarians in practicing these skills. The information in this article relies closely on the work provided through the Bayer Animal Health Communications Project.

Successfully discussing financial issues with clients is integral to delivering optimal patient and client care. Fostering patient health, promoting client satisfaction, and maximizing financial revenues are compatible and attainable goals. Enabling clients to make informed decisions and approaching financial conversations with confidence are rites of passage in the journey toward becoming a true professional.

Given the expectations of clients and the resultant impact of end-of-life conversations on pet owners and the veterinary team, compassionate end-of-life communication is considered to be an ethical obligation, a core clinical skill, and integral to the success of a veterinary team. End-of-life communication is related to significant clinical outcomes, including enduring veterinarian-client-patient relationships and veterinarian and client satisfaction. Effective techniques for end-of-life communication can be taught and are a series of learned skills. The purpose of this article is to present best practices for delivering bad news and euthanasia decision-making discussions. In this article, the SPIKES six-step model (setting, perception, invitation, knowledge, empathize, and summarize) currently employed in medical curricula is utilized to structure end-of-life conversations in veterinary medicine.

Veterinarians working in emergency situations are frequently faced with challenging communication situations. Obtaining informed consent is often difficult because of the emotional content of the situation and the limited amount of time available. Emergency veterinarians are also frequently required to deliver bad, sad, or unwelcome news to clients. Using effective communication skills in these situations may decrease the anxiety and stress for the health care team and contribute to several positive outcomes for the client.

Although the term *compassion fatigue* is often used interchangeably with the term *burnout,* they are two different concepts. Compassion fatigue stems from an overcommitment to work that involves caring for others and is considered by some to be a kind of secondary posttraumatic stress disorder. Because they often invest themselves deeply in the animals they care for, veterinarians, technicians, and other members of an animal health team may be particularly vulnerable to compassion fatigue. This article summarizes the current state of knowledge about compassion fatigue, describes its symptoms, and suggests ways to prevent or overcome it.

Disappointing experiences are not uncommon in the increasingly complex setting of veterinary practice. Managing these situations requires that health care teams be sensitive to client disappointments; accept responsibility for engaging with clients to resolve them; and act ethically, sensitively, and flexibly to reach the best resolutions possible while learning from the experience to reduce the potential for recurrence. The reward for their efforts is an enhanced capability to rebuild rapport, trust, credibility, and loyalty after disappointments and adverse outcomes. Success should translate into a more satisfying practice that builds and maintains its client base and minimizes its liability risks.

Clients may appear compliant but may not fully adhere to recommendations made by the veterinarian or veterinary technician for many reasons. Client adherence is directly related to one's communication skills, which can be practiced by all members of the health care team in each client encounter. The four habits approach to enhancing communication skills has been tested in a large human health care organization and shown to result in greater satisfaction between patients and doctors as well as in improved adherence to recommendations. This model is easily adapted to small animal practice and provides the foundation for a relationship-centered approach to care.

Veterinarians frequently encounter situations that are morally charged and potentially difficult to manage. Situation involving euthanasia, end-of-life care, economics, and inadequate provision of care create practical and moral dilemmas. Ethical tension may be attributable to differences in beliefs regarding the moral value of animals, client and veterinary responsibilities, and deciding what is best for an animal. Veterinarians can employ communication skills used in medical situations to explore the reasons underpinning ethical dilemmas and to search for solutions with clients, staff, and colleagues.

Veterinary professionals must meet the growing expectations of a diverse range of clients to sustain success in veterinary medicine. Few veterinarians, however, receive comprehensive skills training for communicating effectively with clients, particularly among special populations, such as children and older adults. An increasing number of veterinary professionals have recognized a need to master requisite skills for effectively interacting with pet-owning families. This article highlights the importance of the human-animal bond for children and older adults, addresses issues of pet loss, and provides suggestions for meeting the communication needs of both populations.

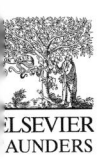

ELSEVIER
SAUNDERS

VETERINARY CLINICS
SMALL ANIMAL PRACTICE

FORTHCOMING ISSUES

March 2007

Clinical Pathology and Diagnostic Techniques
Robin W. Allison, DVM, PhD
and James Meinkoth, DVM, PhD
Guest Editors

May 2007

Evidence-Based Veterinary Medicine
Peggy L. Schmidt, DVM, MS
Guest Editor

July 2007

The Thyroid
Cynthia R. Ward, VMD, PhD
Guest Editor

RECENT ISSUES

November 2006

Dietary Management and Nutrition
Claudia A. Kirk, DVM, PhD
Joseph W. Bartges, DVM, PhD
Guest Editors

September 2006

Current Topics in Clinical Pharmacology and Therapeutics
Dawn Merton Boothe, DVM, PhD
Guest Editor

July 2006

Wound Management
Steven F. Swaim, DVM, MS
D.J. Krahwinkel, DVM, MS
Guest Editors

THE CLINICS ARE NOW AVAILABLE ONLINE!

Access your subscription at:
http://www.theclinics.com

Vet Clin Small Anim 37 (2007) xiii

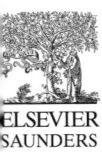

ELSEVIER
SAUNDERS

VETERINARY CLINICS
SMALL ANIMAL PRACTICE

ERRATUM

Feline Diabetes Mellitus: Low Carbohydrates Versus High Fiber?

Claudia A. Kirk, DVM, PhD[a]

[a]Department of Small Animal Clinical Sciences, Veterinary Teaching Hospital, College of Veterinary Medicine, The University of Tennessee, Knoxville, TN 37996-4545, USA

I n the November 2006 issue (volume 36, number 6), on page 1304 of the article "Feline Diabetes Mellitus: Low Carbohydrates Versus High Fiber?" by Claudia A. Kirk, DVM, PhD, there was an error in wording on the second line from the bottom of the page. The full sentence should read, "These are good choices because they are palatable, low in carbohydrates, and fortified with vitamins and minerals that may be beneficial in DM."

0195-5616/07/$ – see front matter
doi:10.1016/j.cvsm.2006.11.010

Vet Clin Small Anim 37 (2007) xv–xvi

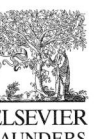

VETERINARY CLINICS
SMALL ANIMAL PRACTICE

Preface

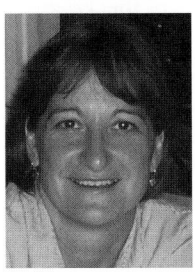 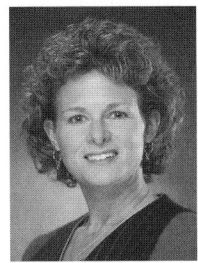 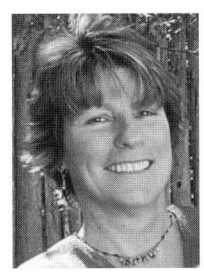

Karen K. Cornell, DVM, PhD
Jennifer C. Brandt, MSW, LISW, PhD
Kathleen A. Bonvicini, MPH

Guest Editors

Veterinarians have long understood the importance of effective communication in our profession. How can we say this with confidence? Because when veterinarians set out to hire veterinary associates, their first question of a referee is often, "Can the applicant talk to people? Will he/she do well with my clients? What are his/her people skills?" Ironically, although veterinarians understand the importance and necessity of communication skills to ensure successful practice, they have long considered learning these skills to be exercises in the "warm and fuzzy" or "touchy feely" category. Assigning such labels to the core skills that comprise effective communication may reflect the discomfort that we as veterinary professionals experience when examining how our interpersonal skills are perceived by others. Such labels may also create barriers to actively engaging in communication skills training. As a profession, we are eager to pursue the latest in "hard" science, eg, diagnostics and therapeutic techniques; however, the best diagnostic and treatment competencies fall short if the ability to relate to clients, colleagues, and staff is lacking. The importance of balancing what has been traditionally known as hard science with communication skills has been underscored since the publication of the KPMG and Brakke studies. These studies have highlighted the importance of integrating communication training throughout all levels of veterinary education. Moreover, there has been a preponderance of research evidence in human medicine that has demonstrated a strong correlation between communication and several healthcare outcomes, including satisfaction, adherence to treatment, malpractice risk, and diagnostic accuracy.

0195-5616/07/$ – see front matter
doi:10.1016/j.cvsm.2006.11.012

The results of these and other studies identify communication skills as a critical skill set that has been lacking in veterinary medical education. What was once considered a "soft" skill is now acknowledged as *essential* to providing high-quality clinical care for our clients and patients. This issue of the *Veterinary Clinics of North America* focuses on the role of communication in the practice of veterinary medicine. It is intended to identify essential communication tools, provide useful examples of how these tools can improve your practice in a variety of contexts, and offer suggestions for the use of such tools within the practice team. It is important to note that the editors and authors of this issue represent an array of disciplines, including veterinary nutrition, large and small animal surgery, critical care, exotic animal medicine, and large animal ambulatory practice. Also included among the authors are experts in the fields of social work, psychology, human medicine, and law—all specialists who work within veterinary settings or who collaborate closely with members of the veterinary profession. We believe that this multidisciplinary approach emphasizes the importance of communication and the need for collaborative approaches across our profession.

Karen K. Cornell, DVM, PhD
Department of Small Animal Medicine and Surgery
College of Veterinary Medicine
University of Georgia
501 South D.W. Brooks Drive
Athens, GA 30602-7390, USA

E-mail address: kcornell@vet.uga.edu

Jennifer C. Brandt, MSW, LISW, PhD
College of Veterinary Medicine
The Ohio State University
601 Vernon Tharp Street
Columbus, OH 43210-1089, USA

E-mail address: honoringthebond@osu.edu

Kathleen A. Bonvicini, MPH
Institute for Healthcare Communication
555 Long Wharf Drive, 13th Floor
New Haven, CT 06511-5901, USA

E-mail address: kbonvicini@healthcarecomm.org

Vet Clin Small Anim 37 (2007) 1–17

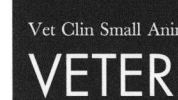

VETERINARY CLINICS
SMALL ANIMAL PRACTICE

It May Be a Dog's Life But the Relationship with Her Owners Is Also Key to Her Health and Well Being: Communication in Veterinary Medicine

Cindy L. Adams, MSW, PhD[a],*, Richard M. Frankel, PhD[b]

[a]Veterinary Medicine-Clinical Communication, Faculty of Veterinary Medicine, University of Calgary, G380, 3330 Hospital Drive, NW Calgary, Alberta T2N 4N1, Canada
[b]Regenstrief Institute, Indiana University School of Medicine, RG-6, 1050 Wishard Boulevard, Indianapolis, IN 46202, USA

I am writing to you, to describe the situation I had to deal with, because I took my dog to Random Animal Hospital. Never have I seen such incompetence. My dog did not receive proper care. It was obvious that this veterinarian wanted nothing more from me than my money and he charged me as much as he could. But, my dog was in worse condition after Dr. X was finished with him that afternoon. And I felt like I was part of a three ring circus, due to the numerous people I didn't even know but had to deal with when I was at the Hospital with Toby. ….This was probably the worst experience I've had in my life.

The excerpt above comes from a review of letters of complaint to the College of Veterinarians of Ontario (CVO). It illustrates one of the most pervasive problems in veterinary practice today: a lack of trust and poor communication that clients experience with veterinary professionals. A recent issue of *Update*, a newsletter published by the CVO, reported that 60% to 67% of complaints from 2002 to 2004 contained some concern regarding communication [1]. A list too extensive to include in this article was published itemizing the most prevalent types of communication problems found in the complaint letters. These included failure to ask for the pet's name, return phone calls, obtain consent, provide postoperative instructions, or demonstrate empathy at the end of a pet's life. Poor communication in human medicine has been associated with higher rates of medication errors, patient dissatisfaction,

---

Parts of this article are identical to that published in a previous communication; Frankel RM. Pets, vets and frets: what relationship-centered care research has to offer veterinary medicine. JVME 2006;33(1):20–7; and are reproduced with permission of the copyright owners of this work.

*Corresponding author. *E-mail address*: cadams@ucalgary.ca (C.L. Adams).

nonadherence, suboptimal biomedical and psychosocial outcomes, and claims for medical malpractice [2].

An emerging line of research in veterinary medicine has begun to investigate the impact of communication on small animal veterinarian–client–patient consultations [3]. Despite obvious differences between human and veterinary medicine, it is clear that there is substantial overlap in the kinds of communication mishaps found in both. Over-reliance on technology, a disease-based approach to training and practice, and pressing economic considerations may result in relationships that fail to meet client expectations.

Problems in communication have been recognized in the practice community and more recently in schools of veterinary medicine. As a result, significant gaps in communication and management skills training for veterinary students have been identified [4,5]. In response to the issues raised by these studies, a consortium of veterinary schools has attempted to define the competencies needed for practice success in veterinary medicine. With the assistance of the organizational consulting firm Personnel Decision International a list of non-technical competencies deemed necessary for practice success was generated. Communication was especially featured [6].

In 2002, Lloyd and Walsh [7] developed a recommended curriculum intended to prepare entry-level graduates for success in practice. In a recent survey by Lloyd and King [8], 23 of the 27 participating veterinary schools in the United States indicated they were making changes to respond to the KPMG study. These changes fell into the categories of admissions, orientation, curriculum, cocurricular, and other. The other category included administrative changes, the development of a combined degree program (such as the DVM-MBA), and training in research. It was also noted that curricular changes were the most widely reported response to the recommendations made by the KPMG study. Targeted additions to the curriculum included team building, business management, marketing, professionalism and interpersonal skills, law/ethics, personal finances, communication, entrepreneurship, and life skills. Although Lloyd and King [8] concluded that "widespread programmatic changes are being implemented in the veterinary schools and colleges" it is not clear exactly what these schools are doing differently and whether they are addressing all of the nontechnical competencies listed or only a select group.

Until recently, communication skills were part of the informal curriculum, learned through practical experience, and without a formal assessment or evaluation process. It seems logical that as the veterinary profession moves to embrace communication skills training in a spectrum of settings from core curricula at veterinary schools to continuing education, efforts should be made to understand the best practices and most effective methods for teaching, learning, and application of communication skills to small and large animal practice settings.

Serious initiatives are underway to provide continuing education on communication topics and skill building for practicing veterinarians. Mega-conferences, including the North American Veterinary Conference, offer a yearly full-day interactive workshop on communication skills for practice. The

American Animal Hospital Association offers a 3-day intensive program for all members of the veterinary team. The emphasis of this program is on team-based communication. Likewise, pharmaceutical and pet food companies recognize the importance of good communication skills and have provided funding for communication research and larger practice initiatives. More recently the National Board of Veterinary Medical Examiners has included assessment of clinical communication skills as part of its examination process for foreign-trained veterinarians.

In this short article, we offer a framework for communicating with clients and colleagues that links elements of communication with processes and outcomes of care. Using excerpts from letters of complaint, we also provide practical examples of how clinical communication skills can lead to more effective client relationships in practice. We also offer our ideas about how to develop an individual communication skills repertoire in practice. Our goal is to add momentum and empiric support for recognizing the importance of practice-level communication skills in achieving successful clinical outcomes.

EVIDENCE-BASED MODEL FOR COMMUNICATING IN PRACTICE

The Four Habits Approach

The Four Habits approach was originally developed to synthesize the literature on patient- and relationship-centered interviewing effectiveness in human medicine. This model is based on what physicians actually do in practice plus additional strategies that they find practical and useful for practice. Relationship-centered care is founded on four principles: (1) relationships should encompass the entire personhood of the participants, (2) emotions are an important part of these relationships, (3) providers and patients can and do influence one another, and (4) forming genuine relationships in health care is morally valuable [9].

The original model, published as a monograph in 1996 and updated in 2003, was designed for educational and research purposes [10,11]. In the time that it has been in use, more than 10,000 physicians have been trained using the approach. The model has been shown to be valid and reliable [12]. Further, there is support to show that physicians trained in the model score higher in patient satisfaction scores for a period of at least 6 months posttraining compared with physicians not trained in this model [13].

It was Aristotle (384 BC–322 BC) who said, "We are what we repeatedly do. Excellence then, is not an act, but a habit." We use the term habit to denote an organized pattern of thinking and acting during the clinical encounter. Much as clinicians use pattern recognition to think about and diagnose disease, the Four Habits—invest in the beginning, elicit the patient's perspective, demonstrate empathy, and invest in the end—provide the background for clinicians to recognize and embody effective communication strategies. The goals of the Four Habits are to establish rapport and build trust rapidly, facilitate the effective exchange of information, demonstrate caring and concern, and increase the likelihood of adherence and positive health outcomes, respectively. In addition to the relevance of the model in human medicine, the Four Habits model has high applicability to veterinary practice.

A growing evidence base suggests that patients and physicians derive considerable satisfaction from interpersonal aspects of care [14]. It also documents that certain clinician behaviors affect the likelihood of achieving desired outcomes or avoiding negative outcomes, such as medical malpractice [15,16]. From an educational perspective there is ample evidence that clinical communication skills can be taught, learned, and practiced [17]. It is our contention that the same increase in satisfaction and successful outcomes with effective communication also holds for veterinary medicine.

Overview of the Approach

The communication tasks that make up the Four Habits are organized into categories of skills, techniques, and payoffs (Table 1). In addition, the habits and associated skills are seen as nested and interrelated. For example, asking an animal owner or agent to share all their concerns at the beginning of a visit, exploring their perspective, and showing appropriate empathy all set the stage for successfully engaging in joint decision making and education.

Habit 1: Invest in the Beginning

Three key skills come into play at the beginning of the client encounter with the practitioner. These are: creating rapport quickly, eliciting the full spectrum of concerns, and planning the visit.

Creating rapport quickly

The first few moments of the veterinary encounter are often treated as small talk and irrelevant to the clinical business at hand. Although this may be true in a narrow technical sense, the opening moments are a gateway for establishing trust and creating a lasting impression of the encounter from a communication perspective.

Once beyond the opening moments and small talk it seems that veterinarians do not use skills, such as open-ended questioning, that are known to create rapport. For example, Shaw and colleagues [3] found that only 7% of veterinarian time was spent gathering data using open-ended questions. The dominant form of question asking in this study was closed ended. This form of inquiry limits a client's ability to respond with additional concerns as the example provided in Box 1 illustrates.

Notice in this example that there is no attempt on the veterinarian's part to join with the client. Instead a series of closed-ended questions has been used to elicit biomedical information. The pattern of questioning limits the owner/client to a series of yes or no replies from which it is difficult to discern if there are any additional concerns. This type of interviewing style is characteristic of a veterinarian-centered approach. In human medicine, this approach is associated with poor adherence, satisfaction, and trust [18,19].

The example in Box 2 illustrates a veterinarian using several Habit 1 skills to elicit the full spectrum of client concerns about the pet. Notice how this line of questioning focuses first on the relationship by inquiring about something shared in the last visit before entering into the business of the current encounter. Addressing the relationship first sets the tone for opening the clinical inquiry about the reason for the pet's visit.

In addition, the veterinarian uses open-ended questions that elicit factual and affective information from the client. The veterinarian also uses a linguistic device known as a re-completer to facilitate the relationship and elicit high-quality clinical information. After the client says "She's just sort of been listless lately," the veterinarian simply repeats a key word, listless, with an upwardly rising intonation. This functions as an invitation to tell the story that is the context for her statement about the pet's condition.

After the patient introduces the story with "Yes, it started about 3 days ago" the veterinarian uses another linguistic device known as a continuer. These are vocalizations, such as "mmh hmh," "go on," "I see," that encourage the speaker to elaborate on the content and emotional impact of what she is saying. In this case, the veterinarian's open-ended continuer produces a statement of concern on the owner/client's part. The veterinarian's silence at this point produces strong affect, as the owner/client asserts: "I'm scared to death that she might have gotten rabies." In developing an approach to the owner/client, this is potentially important information because it provides a convincing rationale for why the owner/client is seeking care for her pet.

There is little time difference between these approaches. In human medicine it takes about 1 minute longer to invest in the relationship and encourage the full expression of concerns than to remain exclusively problem- or disease-focused [20]. The extra minute seems to be time well spent. As a habit of practice one might think about inquiring about and noting something personal in each owner/client's chart after each visit and using it as an opening inquiry in the next visit.

The payoff for Habit 1 is that clients feel welcomed, safe, and listened to, within a framework and organization for the visit that is clear and explicit. The value of this habit in human medicine has been demonstrated in research conducted by the Headache Study Group at the University of Western Ontario [21]. They found that the strongest predictor of resolution of chronic headache symptoms at 1 year follow-up was the perception on the patient's part that the clinician had listened completely to all of their concerns in the first visit. Investing in the beginning sets the stage and tone and provides the plan for the rest of the visit.

Habit 2: Elicit the Owner's/Client's Perspective

In human medicine, the current climate of consumer demand for high-quality care and information, ethical and legal standards requiring that patients be fully informed, and increasing concern about poor communication as a source of medical errors all point to the importance of eliciting the patient's perspective. As recently as July 2006, an Institute of Medicine report on medication errors noted the critical importance of a paradigm shift from doctor-centered to patient- and relationship-centered communication stating that "one of the most effective ways to reduce medication errors is to move toward a model of health care where there is more of a partnership between the patients and the health care providers" [22].

Table 1
The Four Habits Model adapted for veterinary medicine

Habit	Skills	Techniques and examples	Payoff
Invest in the beginning	Create rapport quickly Elicit client's concerns Plan the visit with the client	Introduce self Acknowledge wait Convey knowledge of patient's history by commenting on prior visit or problem Attend to patient/client comfort Make a social comment or ask a nonmedical question to put client at ease Adapt own language, pace, and posture in response to client Start with open-ended questions: "What would you like help with today?" "I understand that you're here for … Could you tell me more about that ?" "What else?" Speak directly with client when using an interpreter Repeat concerns back to check understanding Let client know what to expect: "How about if we start with talking more about…, then I'll do an exam, and then we'll go over possible tests/ways to treat this? Sound OK?" Prioritize when necessary: "Let's make sure we talk about X and Y. It sounds like you also want to make sure we cover Z. If we can't get to the other concerns, let's…"	Establishes a welcoming atmosphere Allows faster access to real reason for visit Increases diagnostic accuracy Requires less work Minimizes "Oh, by the way…" at the end of visit Facilitates negotiating an agenda Decreases potential for conflict

Elicit the patient's perspective	Ask for client's ideas Elicit specific requests Explore the impact on the patient/client's life	Assess client's point of view: "What do you think is causing your symptoms?" "What worries you most about this problem?" Ask about ideas from significant others Determine client's goal in seeking care: "When you've been thinking about this visit, how were you hoping I could help?" Check context: "How has the illness affected daily activities?"	Respects diversity Allows client to provide important diagnostic clues Uncovers hidden concerns Reveals use of alternative treatments or requests for tests Improves diagnosis of depression and anxiety
Demonstrate empathy	Be open to client's emotions Make at least one empathic statement Convey empathy nonverbally Be aware of your own reactions	Assess changes in body language and voice tone Look for opportunities to use brief empathic comments or gestures Name a likely emotion: "That sounds really upsetting." Compliment patient on efforts to address problem Use a pause, touch, or facial expression Use own emotional response as a clue to what client might be feeling Take a brief break if necessary	Adds depth and meaning to the visit Builds trust, leading to better diagnostic information, adherence, and outcomes Makes limit-setting or saying "no" easier

(continued on next page)

Table 1 (continued)			
Habit	**Skills**	**Techniques and examples**	**Payoff**
Invest in the end	Deliver diagnostic information Provide education Involve client in making decisions Complete the visit	Frame diagnosis in terms of client's original concerns Test client's comprehension Explain rationale for tests and treatments Review possible side effects and expected course of recovery Recommend lifestyle changes Provide written materials and refer to other sources Discuss treatment goals Explore options, listening for the client's preferences Set limits respectfully: "I can understand how getting that test makes sense to you. From my point of view, since the results won't help us diagnose or treat the symptoms, I suggest we consider this instead." Assess client's ability and motivation to carry out plan Ask for additional questions: "What questions do you have?" Assess satisfaction: "Did you get what you needed?" Reassure client of ongoing care	Increases potential for collaboration Influences health outcomes Improves adherence Reduces return calls and visits Encourages self care

Adapted from Frankel RM, Stein T, Krupat E. The four habits approach to effective clinical communication. Oakland, CA: Kaiser Permanente; 2003. p. 17; with permission.

Box 1: Opening the visit: closed questioning

Vet: Hello Ms. Jones. What problems is Fluffy having?
Owner: She's just sort of been listless lately.
Vet: When did it begin?
Owner: It started about 3 days ago.
Vet: What was going on then?
Owner: She was out in the back yard chasing squirrels and when she came back in she just went to her bed and laid down. She's been sort of listless ever since.
Vet: Has she been eating okay?
Owner: I think so.
Vet: Any coughing or vomiting?
Owner: No.
Vet: Going to the bathroom regularly?
Owner: Yes
Vet: Noticed any loose stool?
Owner: No.

Although acknowledged as important to the care process, many physicians, and veterinarians do not avail themselves of the opportunity to build partnerships during the interview. Such missed opportunities relate to increased nonadherence and medication errors. A study by Braddock and coworkers [23] found that only one in five primary care physicians and surgeons inquired about the perspectives of their patients. According to the authors the rationale for exploring patient perspectives is that "Physicians may assume that patients will speak up if they disagree with a decision, but patients often need to be

Box 2: Using open-ended questions to build relationships

Vet: Hi Ms. Jones. It's good to see you again. How have you been since I saw you last? I seem to remember that you were just leaving to go visit your daughter in Holland. How was your visit with her?
Owner: Oh it was marvelous. Thanks for asking!
Vet: Sure, and how is Fluffy doing since she was here last?
Owner: She's just sort of been listless lately.
Vet: Listless?
Owner: Yes it started about 3 days ago.
Vet: Mmh hmh.
Owner: She was out in the back yard chasing squirrels and when she came back in she just went to her bed and laid down. She's been sort of listless ever since.
Vet: Mmh hmh.
Owner: You know it's really concerning to me.
Vet: (Silence)
Owner: I'm just scared to death that she might have gotten rabies and might have to be put down or something like that.
Vet: I can see that you're concerned and I'll come back to that in a moment. Before I do is there anything else you're concerned about?
Owner: No.

asked for their opinion. It should be clear to the patient [and the pet owner] that it is appropriate to disagree or ask for more time" [23]. For example, asking "Does that sound reasonable?" or "What do you think?" invites patients or clients to share their views.

Habit 2 serves several important functions: showing respect for the client's experience and individuality, developing partnerships, and comparing similarities and differences in understanding. Early work by Pantell and colleagues [24] in pediatrics showed that children who have asthma have their own needs, and addressing these can improve their satisfaction and adherence to treatment. A similar finding was recently reported by Staiger and colleagues [25], who studied low back pain in adults.

In everyday life, owner/clients frequently engage in a process similar to differential diagnosis. That is, they exclude certain causes and explanations for their observations and include others. Knowing specifically what meaning they are giving to their animals' symptoms allows the practitioner to frame the rest of the dialog accordingly. For example, the owner in the second example (Box 2), who was "scared to death," may seem unusually worried about symptoms that seem vague or minimal to the practitioner. Finding out the client's attribution or source of concern by eliciting the client's perspective often clarifies the situation and offers an opportunity to strengthen the relationship. The following excerpts from letters of complaint serve to highlight the impact of missed opportunities to determine the client's perspective.

Letter 1

> I am writing this letter to lodge a formal complaint against Dr. X. Our dog was assessed by Dr. X for dental health. He advised us to get Peppy's teeth cleaned and possibly there would be some extractions of teeth due to bad gums. Dr. X removed 12 teeth during the cleaning! Later on he removed another 7 teeth. He did not have permission to take our dog's teeth out. Now we have to water down his food so he can eat and he has to eat on one side of his mouth. Did our dog really need 19 teeth taken out? Dr. X did renovations to his clinic about a year ago. Could there be any connection?
>
> —Yours sincerely, The client

Letter 2

> "On January 3rd, a week after Mitsy's next heat had finished we noticed she was drinking large amounts of water again. We called ABC Animal Hospital on January 5 and I explained my concerns to Sue, the receptionist (as well as Mitsy's recent history at the Hospital). An appointment was made to have her looked at. The blood tests from last May were sent to the hospital as well. During the week Mitsy was eating on and off but still energetic. Both my wife and I felt blood work and X-rays were needed based on what we had learned at the previous hospital. After the examination we all agreed that Mitsy should be spayed and we booked an appointment. We were surprised that no baseline diagnostics were taken given our

> description of the symptoms that we reviewed with the Dr. We were told instead that they like to do the tests the day of the operation. We left the hospital intending to return the following week for the surgery. We were given no indication that we needed to be concerned about infection or pyometra, even though she had a recent heat. ... The ovariohysterectomy was performed the following week. We went to see Mitsy that evening. We were told that Mitsy's uterus has been infected and there were concerns about her condition. We mentioned to the person we were seeing that she had an exam the previous week and even though we requested tests at that time we were told to wait until today. Mitsy had to stay for the night. The following day the Dr. contacted us and told us she had septicemia and we should come right over. We stayed to comfort her for 3 hours and until she passed away. All the vets were out of the clinic for lunch when she died. A Dr. had to be called back to the clinic to pronounce her dead. He told us it was a closed pyometra that induced the sepsis and loss of life. We are still in shock over her loss and feel that if proper tests were done and action taken, she would still be alive today. She did not deserve to die this way.
> —Sincerely, Client

In human medicine Tuckett and coworkers [26] found that patients who were able to fully explain their illnesses to their physician recalled more information and were more committed to treatment. In addition to better adherence to treatment recommendations, another payoff for Habit 2 is learning about how owner/clients view the health, illness, and disease of their pets. This information is valuable in considering how best to communicate prognostic and treatment information to owner/clients and family members. In the case above, had the veterinarian attempted to build a partnership with the owner by explaining that there was a relatively low likelihood of a serious underlying problem requiring immediate testing, the decision not to test would have been shared rather than perceived as unilateral. Although the outcome would not have changed, the owner's perception of neglect on the part of the veterinarian might have been different.

Habit 3: Demonstrate Empathy

Caring and compassion have characterized the relationship of human and animal healers to their clients for centuries. In the modern era, great technological advances and economic pressures have led to a relative de-emphasis on the therapeutic benefits of caring and compassion in training and practice. Research in human and veterinary medicine has found low levels of empathy expressed during visits. For instance, Shaw and colleagues [3] found empathy expressed in only 7% of the 300 companion animal appointments they studied. Suchman and colleagues [27] found an even lower level of empathy in their qualitative study of empathy in human medicine. Researchers have linked the presence or absence of caring to a range of outcomes, including satisfaction, adherence to medical recommendations, and propensity to sue [28].

If caring and compassion form the core conceptual basis of the healing relationship, empathy is the core skill for enacting it (see Table 1). Although understood to be therapeutic, empathy does not occur often in clinical encounters [3,27]. One barrier to its use is the perception of limited time availability to do anything but the most instrumental clinical tasks in the visit. Many clinicians assume that it is not possible to demonstrate empathy under such time-limited circumstances. Contrary to this belief, researchers studying an elite group of outstanding clinicians observed that they invariably found a way to respond to patient emotion using windows of opportunity, selectively attending to moments in the encounter that seemed to get to the heart of their patients' concerns [29]. Other research supports the notion that a patient's appreciation of an empathic response is sustaining to the clinician and adds meaning and depth to the relationship [30].

Accurately identifying emotions depends on observing nonverbal behavior, such as facial expression and body posture, and listening closely to the patient or client's tone of voice as he or she describes the experience. In human medicine, physicians who are sensitive to nonverbal expression of emotion have more satisfied patients [31]. Likewise, physicians who use eye contact appropriately are more likely to detect and treat emotional distress [32]. There is also evidence, based on content-filtered speech, that voice tone is a reliable predictor of follow up to treatment recommendations [33].

In a study of referrals for treatment of alcohol abuse, a warm accepting tone of voice on the provider's part was highly associated with follow-up from the referral [33]. In a recent study using specialized analysis of content-filtered speech, Ambady and colleagues [15] were successfully able to distinguish between surgeons who had never been sued and those who had been sued for malpractice at least twice.

Often patients or clients only hint at an emotion. Statements such as "Fluffy seems listless," or "What do you think about surgery for Fluffy's cancer?" do not express an emotion directly. Suchman and coworkers [27] defined these occurrences as potential empathic opportunities (PEOs) and suggested that they are often used by patients to test whether it is safe to talk about the underlying emotion. Clinicians who attend to emotional clues and cues improve the quality of communication and relationships with patients. Likewise, Suchman and coworkers [27] noted that when emotional clues are ignored, patients will repeat or escalate their concerns or surface them only at the end of the visit.

In the following excerpt from a letter of complaint to the CVO, a client's experience of lack of empathy is compounded by the more routine aspects of handling animals following death and the business side of practice:

> On Friday morning I received a phone call from the veterinary clinic telling me that Sasha was not well and I should come to the clinic as soon as possible. She told me she might not make it. I had promised Sasha if she was ever to leave this earth I would be with her to show my immense love for her. I had just come from the shower to get the phone. I promptly threw on my clothes and drove there. She had died before I arrived and was brought to me in a box. Only minutes later both the Dr. and the technician were both very interested in selling me a plot of land to bury her and to sell me a gravestone to commemorate her. Before I left to bury my beloved

> Sasha, and I was crying profusely, the technician had the utter audacity, gall and disrespect to ask me what I would like to do with my invoice!

Helping owners/clients move from hinting at an emotion to its full expression is part of the work of empathy. Cohen-Cole [34] identified five types of verbal statements that convey empathy and suggested a generic format for each. They are:

> Reflection—"It sounds like you're concerned that Fluffy ..."
> Legitimization—"Anyone would feel scared ..."
> Support—"I will be there for you no matter what happens ..."
> Partnership—"I think we can figure this out together ..."
> Respect—"I have confidence that you'll do the right thing ..."

In addition, the use of nonverbal actions, such as silence, touch, gaze, facial expression, and body posture, are all associated with conveying empathy. The payoff for demonstrating empathy is getting to the heart of the problem and relieving emotional distress [35]. Had the technician described in the letter above responded to the client's strong emotion by demonstrating empathy the technician would in all likelihood have found the client more than willing to settle her account after a brief opportunity to adjust to her beloved pet's death.

Empathy adds depth and meaning to the relationship and also builds trust. When the time comes to make difficult or complex decisions, having explored the emotional terrain surrounding the issue facilitates partnerships and informed decision making. Poignant to veterinary practice is the issue of costs. Hardee and colleagues [35] describe skills necessary for talking about cost with patients including the use of "we" statements and "I wish ..." as a platform for shared decision making and a search for alternative approaches or plans [36]. Timing the discussion of services and costs so that they occur after empathy has been demonstrated in the face of strong client emotion ensures that subsequent discussions will take place within a trustworthy affective partnership.

Habit 4: Invest in the End

Although the first three Habits are based on gathering information, Habit 4, investing in the end, is primarily focused on information sharing. This is reflected in the tasks at the end of the encounter, namely, delivering diagnostic information, encouraging participation in decision making, and checking for understanding of recommended treatments. Communicating bad news and its effects on family members can be a real challenge. Although it may be required in practice, many physicians receive no formal training in this area as the following narrative from a senior physician recounting his training experience in delivering bad news attests:

> I was a third year student on an ER rotation when a family (grandmother, 10-year-old girl, uncle of girl) came in badly burned in a house fire. The girl was in arrest and despite all efforts died. The grandmother was alive but critically burned. The smell of charred flesh was overpowering. I was sent to ask the mother for an autopsy. Instead of beginning by informing

her of the death I began with: "Sorry to bother you at this time but ..." and
then asked her my question. She screamed and collapsed, hysterical at my
feet. I was aghast, guilty, stunned, felt inadequate to make any appropriate
response. I still feel awful about it to this day.

The costs of poor training in this area are most obvious on the patient side,
although the literature suggests that physicians who make mistakes of this sort
suffer also [37]. Poor outcomes and emotional wounds are a prescription for
patient dissatisfaction and malpractice suits.

The following excerpt from a letter of complaint highlights the client's experience of not having adequate information to make an informed decision about
how to proceed with the care and treatment of her pet:

In September our dog was taken to see Dr. Y because of a lump in the tummy
area. She had a mast cell tumor. Dr. Y advised that the cytology report was
very good and that she could undergo the removal of this tumor with no complications. Rumour came through the surgery with no complications and the
Dr. said she was confident that she had removed it all. We must state that at the
time of this operation under no circumstances did the Dr. discuss with us any
follow-up chemotherapy or preventative measures for prevention of further tu-
mors from developing. We had NO idea there were any such measures available. A year later another lump was discovered in the same area and we took
her back to the same Dr. No labs tests were performed and we were informed
that Rumour was in good shape and could withstand another surgery. ...
Upon our arrival to pick Rumour up after this second surgery she was brought
to us by a technician. She told us that we should immediately upon our arrival
home give our dog a bath in the bathtub and then treat her stitches with hydro-
gen peroxide and water so she would not get infected. We were not informed
when to bring her back to have her stitches removed and she was not given
antibiotics or pain medication. We did as we were told and my husband
bathed the dog ...

The importance of checking for client comprehension and coming to a mutually agreed-upon plan cannot be overemphasized. In addition to shared
decision making and increased adherence to follow-up, using this approach
provides an ideal opportunity to educate clients about their pet's condition
and to correct any misunderstandings or misapprehensions. Grueninger and
coworkers [38] suggest several helpful questions for use in optimizing comprehension and agreement. These include:

After having discussed the various options with you is there anything that I've
    missed or anything that we need to clarify?
Are you comfortable with the plan we've outlined?
Is there anything that would make it difficult or impossible for you to follow the plan?

The payoffs from using Habit 4 are increased collaboration in decision making and a corresponding reduction in risk for error and nonadherence. Further,
focusing on comprehension of diagnostic news, instructions, and recommendations, and barriers to adherence improves alignment between the health care

provider and desired outcomes of care. Finally, knowing how to sensitively deliver bad news can relieve unnecessary suffering on the client's part and make the practice of veterinary medicine more deeply satisfying.

SUMMARY

We have reviewed more than four decades of research and evidence in human medicine that has consistently demonstrated that communication and relationship building impact the quality and outcomes of care. There is emerging evidence in veterinary medicine that many of the same challenges exist in providing clinical care for pets, who cannot speak for themselves, and their owners, who can and do. It seems that improved communication with pet owners is associated with fewer complaints, higher levels of satisfaction, and reductions in medication and other types of errors.

Growing recognition of the benefits of communication skills training has led veterinary medical educators to develop explicit curricula based on evidence of best practices. In doing so they have acknowledged that these skills belong in the formal curriculum and need to be taught just as doing accurate diagnosis and treatment are. As a result, we can expect that the next generations of veterinarians will possess outstanding skills in communicating with their clients.

What can veterinarians do to improve their communication skills in practice? Several options currently exist:

Attend a national meeting in which workshops on communication skills are offered.

Attend an intensive training course on communication skills offered by regional or national organizations. (In human medicine the American Academy on Communication in Healthcare and the European Association for Communication in Healthcare offer 1-, 2.5-, and 5-day intensive courses on improving communication skills. Veterinarians have been active in both organizations.)

Contact the Institute for Healthcare Communication and learn about continuing education opportunities on communication.

Assess your own communication skills using the Four Habits or an equivalent approach. This might include having a colleague observe you for a clinic session and provide feedback on your communication skills. Self-assessment is another possibility.

Use letters of complaint and also those that complement the practice to work on ways to improve communication and relationships with clients and within the health care team.

Partner with one or more colleagues to discuss challenging cases and innovative approaches to communicating more effectively.

Improved communication skills are of demonstrated benefit to clients, but the evidence is that practitioners benefit also. An emphasis on the bottom line may leave veterinarians feeling stressed and demoralized. Investing in habits of practice that result in improved relationships has the added benefit of reminding us of why we went into our chosen fields in the first place and restoring the sense of joy in serving others and alleviating suffering.

References

[1] Robinson R. College of Veterinarians of Ontario (CVO). 2005;21(3):8–9.

[2] Silverman J, Kurtz S, Draper J. Skills for communicating with patients. 2nd edition. Abingdon, Oxon, UK: Radcliffe Medical Press; 2005.

[3] Shaw J, Adams C, Bonnett B, et al. Use of the Roter interaction analysis system to analyze veterinarian-client-patient communication in companion animal practice. J Am Vet Med Assoc 2004;225:222–9.

[4] Brown JP, Silverman JD. The current and future market for veterinarians and veterinary medical services in the United States. J Am Vet Med Assoc 1999;215:161–83.

[5] Cron WL, Slocum JV Jr, Goodnight DB, et al. Executive summary of the Brakke management and behavior study. J Am Vet Med Assoc 2000;217:332–8.

[6] Lewis RE, Klausner JS. Nontechnical competencies underlying career success as a veterinarian. J Am Vet Med Assoc 2003;222:1690–6.

[7] Lloyd J, Walsh DA. Template for a recommended curriculum in veterinary professional development and career success. J Vet Med Educ 2002;29:84–93.

[8] Lloyd J, King LJ. What are the veterinary schools and colleges doing to improve the nontechnical skills, knowledge, aptitudes, and attitudes of veterinary students? J Am Vet Med Assoc 2004;224:1923–4.

[9] Beach MC, Inui TS. Relationship centered care: a constructive reframing. J Gen Intern Med 2006;21S:3–8.

[10] Frankel RM, Stein T, Krupat E. The four habits approach to effective clinical communication. Oakland, CA: Kaiser Permanente; 2003.

[11] Frankel RM, Stein T. The four habits of highly effective clinicians. The Permanente Journal 1999;3(3):79–88.

[12] Krupat E, Frankel RM, Stein T. The four habits coding scheme: validation of an instrument to assess clinicians' communication behaviour. Patient Educ Couns 2006;62(1):38–45.

[13] Stein T, Frankel RM, Krupat E. Enhancing clinician communication skills in a large healthcare organization: a longitudinal case study. Patient Educ Couns 2005;58:4–12.

[14] Arborelius E, Bremberg S. What can doctors do to achieve a successful consultation? Videotaped interviews analyzed by the "consultation map" method. Fam Pract 1992;9:61–6.

[15] Ambady N, Laplante D, Nguyen T, et al. Surgeons' tone of voice: a clue to malpractice history. Surgery 2002;132:5–9.

[16] Levinson W, Roter DL, Mullooly JP, et al. The relationship with malpractice claims among primary care physicians and surgeons. JAMA 1997;277:553–9.

[17] Kurtz S, Silverman J, Draper D. Teaching and learning communication skills in medicine. 2nd edition. Abingdon, Oxon, UK: Radcliffe Medical Press; 2005.

[18] Henbest RJ, Stewart M. Patient-centredness in the consultation, 1. A method of measurement. Fam Pract 1990a;6:249–53.

[19] Henbest RJ, Stewart M. Patient-centredness in the consultation, 2. Does it really make a difference? Fam Pract 1990b;7:28–33.

[20] Stewart M, Brown J, Weston W. Patient-centered interviewing: five provocative questions. Can Fam Physician 1989;35:159–61.

[21] Headache Study Group. Predictors of outcome in patients presenting to family physicians: a one year prospective study. Headache 1986;26:285–94.

[22] Committee on identifying and preventing medication errors. In: Aspden P, Wolcott J, Bottman JL, et al, editors. Washington, DC: National Academic Press; 2007.

[23] Braddock CH, Edwards KA, Hasenberg NM, et al. Informed decision making in outpatient practice: time to get back to basics. JAMA 1999;282:2313–20.

[24] Pantell RH, Stewart TJ, Dias JK, et al. Physician communication with children and parents. Pediatrics 1982;70:396–402.

[25] Staiger TO, Jravik JG, Deyo RA, et al. Patient physician agreement as a predictor of outcomes in patients with back pain. J Gen Intern Med 2005;20:935–7.

[26] Tuckett D, Boulton M, Olson C, et al. Meetings between experts: An approach to sharing ideas among medical experts. London: Tavistock; 1985.

[27] Suchman AL, Markakis K, Beckman HB, et al. A model of empathic communication in the medical interview. JAMA 1997;277:678–82.

[28] Lester GW, Smith SG. Listening and talking to patients: a remedy for malpractice suits? West J Med 1993;158:268–72.

[29] Branch WT, Malik TK. Using "windows of opportunities" in brief interviews to understand patients' concerns. JAMA 1993;269:1667–8.

[30] Horowitz CR, Suchman AS, Branch W, et al. What do doctors find meaningful about their work? Ann Intern Med 2003;138:772–6.

[31] DiMatteo MR, Taranta A, Friedman HS, et al. Predicting patient satisfaction from physicians' nonverbal communication skills. Med Care 1980;18:376–87.

[32] Goldberg DP, Steele JJ, Smith C, et al. Training family doctors to recognize psychiatric illness with increased accuracy. Lancet 1980;2:521–3.

[33] Milmoe S, Rosenthal R, Blane HT, et al. The doctor's voice: postdictor of successful referral of alcoholic patients. J Abnorm Psychol 1967;72:78–84.

[34] Cohen-Cole SA. The medical interview: the three function approach. St. Louis, MO: Mosby/Yearbook; 1991. p. 21–27.

[35] Hardee JY, Platt FW, Kasper IK. Discussing health care costs with patients: an opportunity for empathic communication. J Gen Intern Med 2005;20:666–9.

[36] Tennstedt SL. Empowering older patients to communicate more effectively in the medical encounter. In: Adelman R, Greene MG, editors. Clinics in geriatrics medicine: communication between older patients and their physicians. Philadelphia: W.B. Saunders; 2000. p. 61–70.

[37] Christensen JF, Levinson W, Dunn PM. The heart of darkness: the impact of perceived mistakes on physicians. J Gen Intern Med 1992;7:424–31.

[38] Grueninger UJ, Duffy D, Goldstein MG. Patient education in the medical encounter: how to facilitate learning, behavior change, and coping. In: Lipkin MJ, Putnam SM, Lazare A, editors. The medical interview. New York: Springer-Verlag; 1995. p. 129–33.

Vet Clin Small Anim 37 (2007) 19–35

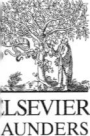

VETERINARY CLINICS
SMALL ANIMAL PRACTICE

The Veterinary Health Care Team: Going from Good to Great

Kathleen L. Ruby, MEd, PhD[a,b,*],
Richard M. DeBowes, DVM, MS[a]

[a]External Relations and Development, Veterinary Clinical Sciences, College of Veterinary Medicine, Washington State University, P.O. Box 646610, Pullman, WA 99164-6610, USA
[b]Department of Counseling, Wellness and Leadership, College of Veterinary Medicine, Washington State University, P.O. Box 647010, Pullman, WA 99164-7010, USA

> Never doubt that a small group of thoughtful, committed people can change the world. Indeed, it is the only thing that ever has. —Margaret Mead
>
> A team is like having a baby tiger given to you at Christmas. It does a wonderful job of keeping the mice away for about 12 months and then it starts to eat the kids. —Anonymous Team Leader, American President Lines

C reating an effective medical team can be one of the major challenges of a veterinarian's professional life. As these two quotes illustrate, working with a team can be either (or both) an exhilarating or distressing undertaking.

Although schooling and training do a great job preparing veterinary professionals with the necessary skills and competencies to practice medicine, almost no consideration is given to teaching the practical proficiencies of hiring, training, and maintaining a group of employees who compose the foundation and scaffolding of a veterinary practice. Teamwork does not automatically occur because people work in the same place. It relies heavily on several factors. These include the group's willingness to cooperate toward shared goals, which involve caring for patients and clients, avoiding costly medical errors, and creating an environment conducive to the well-being of the staff and the clientele.

To reach these goals, it is imperative to discover guiding principles to illuminate the course that must be undertaken. In his influential work *The Seven Habits of Highly Effective People* leadership guru Stephen Covey [1] cited the first two habits for success as being proactive and beginning with the end in mind. The end goal, in this case, is to foster a strong health care team culture. Such

*Corresponding author. Department of Wellness and Leadership, College of Veterinary Medicine, Washington State University, P.O. Box 647010, Pullman, WA 99164-7010.
E-mail address: kruby@vetmed.wsu.edu (K.L. Ruby).

0195-5616/07/$ – see front matter
doi:10.1016/j.cvsm.2006.10.004

results necessitate a clear, hard look at personal biases, negative preconceived notions, or past experiences with teams that may serve to undermine what is possible through wise team leadership. Successful health care teams are like all human relationships. They are possible but they take discernment, desire, and dedication to bring them to fruition.

A CLEAR VISION

Beginning with the end in mind means veterinarians and practice leaders need to take the time to create a clear picture of what their highly functioning health care team would look like and be willing to invest the time, money, and attention needed to make that vision a reality. This process is often a major challenge. Although a well-functioning team with clear roles and strong interpersonal skills will contribute to practice heartiness and provide the DVM and the staff with better working conditions, finding and taking the time to focus on team development is difficult and costly.

If true health care teams are so difficult and time consuming to assemble, why make the effort? A major study in human health care provides a plethora of reasons backed by solid research [2]. In their 2000 study, Kohn and colleagues [2] found that medical errors often occurred because of breakdowns in communication and follow-up between members of a hospital or medical team. This breakdown occurred at all levels and stages of patient care, including misunderstandings about diagnosis and test results and errors in dosing or method of using a drug. Errors occur most commonly because of people system breakdowns, which translate to mean malfunctioning medical teams.

This same study reports that the Institute of Medicine began to look at the reasons for the high rate of medical errors in the United States early in 1999. They estimated that at least 44,000 people and perhaps as many as 98,000 people die in hospitals each year as a result of medical errors that were preventable. In addition to loss of lives, the impact from medical errors produces a cascade of demoralization throughout the health care industry. The acknowledgment of this reality erodes the trust and credibility society places in its medical practitioners. Malpractice costs and awards skyrocket. Patients suffer needlessly. What about the cost to medical teams? These findings undercut the very foundation of medical ethics and the medical calling. One of the primary edicts guiding medical care is "first, do no harm." Health care professionals and their teams pay for these errors with a loss of self-efficacy, morale, and job satisfaction, and increased levels of frustration.

Although similar studies in veterinary health care have not yet been done, it would be prudent for the animal health industry to take note of these findings as studies of medical error in human medicine most likely have their parallels in veterinary medicine. What do researchers suspect is at the root of these types of errors that seem so frighteningly prevalent in medicine today?

COMMUNICATION ROADBLOCKS

A study in the British Medical Journal [3] reaffirms that the communication patterns and behaviors among medical staff contributed greatly to the inefficiencies and errors seen in medical settings. In a hectic office or hospital, medical personnel may become caught up in the task of the moment and fail to consider the larger context of care and how best to share information or solicit assistance when needed. This type of single-mindedness can lead to medical errors, poor attention to patients and clients, and interpersonal aggravation. This same study described how the constant "stops and starts" of verbal interruptions by team members during patient care most likely contribute to reduced levels of care. These interruptions were symptomatic of the lack of awareness group members may have for the work being done outside of their own sphere.

When poor communication is blamed as one of the main culprits contributing to medical error, this is not simply a result of the inadequate transmission of information between two or more people. The failures of adequate communication are often a complex mix of perceived hierarchical differences, contradictory and ambiguous roles, interpersonal power differentials, and conflict between individuals or groups [4]. With evidence pointing to the medical and psychologic costs attributed to poor communications in a medical team, it is apparent that attention to the cultivation of healthy team dynamics would pay many dividends throughout all aspects of practice.

TEAMS DEFINED

Several national studies have indicated that the skills needed to successfully establish and run a viable practice must become part of the DVM's professional repertoire if veterinary clinics are to thrive and flourish. [5,6,7] Most practice owners and associates know when they see a successful team yet are not sure how to describe it or replicate it. To better quantify what is meant by team excellence, it is helpful to examine what business and group research can teach us about building and leading winning teams. What does a successful work team look like and how does it function?

GROUPS OR TEAMS?

It is first important to realize that not all work groups are teams. Let us first examine the difference between the two.

Work groups are coworkers who work together but do not necessarily collaborate in the completion of their job duties. Each member of a work group has a defined set of tasks or responsibilities and these tasks are overseen jointly by the practice manager or leader and the employee. The employee views his or her job in terms of completing or maintaining these tasks. Work planning and execution happens primarily between the employee and the manager. This type of work arrangement works best when the job to be accomplished is simple and repetitive and does not require much between-employee coordination.

Teams, on the other hand, fill a more complicated niche. To work smoothly, a team is composed of a group of individuals united in their professional purpose, values, and vision. Further, they understand that team success depends on their ability to collaborate. They know the complexity and intricate nature of their work depends on not only their own but also their coworkers' efforts and contributions. Team members depend on one another to carry out their jobs and each member must have a sense of how his or her role supports and contributes to the ultimate mission of the workplace. In contrast to the work group, a team joins forces to get the job done and pools their resources to make judicious decisions. They are united in their purpose and understand that their individual jobs are all part of a larger picture [8]. The complex nature of a veterinary medical practice makes it clear that offices should be staffed by teams rather than work groups.

NECESSARY ELEMENTS FOR SUCCESSFUL TEAMS

In his book *Leading Teams: Setting the Stage for Great Performances*, J. Richard Hackman [9] outlines four distinctive elements that contribute to the formation of a successful team: "a team task, clear boundaries, clearly specified authority to manage their own work processes, and membership stability over time" [9]. When these features are in place, teams have the structure and the freedom to adapt to and meet the daily work flow. They also develop a sense of interpersonal rhythm with one another that allows them to communicate clearly and concisely without wasted effort or hierarchical disputes.

There are multiple tasks that must be provided by the team. These include the provision of a high standard of patient and client care, a pleasing and hygienic medical environment, appropriate client-centered atmosphere, efficient office flow, complete and thorough medical record keeping, and a stable and pleasant working environment. These multifaceted tasks necessitate a team of veterinary professionals who practice a high degree of interdependence and joint problem solving. Responsibility extends beyond each individual and the staff must be united in their practice philosophy and vision. Working collaboratively as a team rather than as individuals in a work group provides the structure within which these complex interactions can take place. Management consultant Patrick Lencioni stated that "Teamwork remains the one sustainable competitive advantage that has been largely untapped. I can say confidently that teamwork is almost always lacking within organizations that fail and often present within those that succeed" [10].

Most veterinary practices, on conducting an honest self and team assessment, discover they function not as an actual team, but as a group of individuals working side by side—a work group. If medical care and improved workplace climates are the true aim for our standard of care, we must learn to shift our work groups into the active team model.

THE IMPORTANCE OF THE RIGHT TEAM MEMBERS

Before we discuss how to introduce the conceptualization of health care team within the practice environment, we will delve more deeply into the elements of a team and tasks of the team leader.

First, it is imperative to take stock of how the team is currently functioning. A leader must appraise to what extent the team shares common goals, along with rewards and responsibilities for achieving them. Are individual goals in alignment with the practice goals and the practice mission? Do team members set aside their individual or personal needs for the greater good of the group [10]?

In his book *Good to Great* Jim Collins [11] uses an interesting metaphor to explore the concept of goals and mission. He compares the process of establishing practice purpose or mission as akin to figuring out where the "bus [practice] is going" [11]. Using that analogy, Collins recommended surveying office staff to assess whether the right people are "on the bus" and "in the right seats" [11]. A practice leader, along with the team, needs to strive for clarity in this regard. Although most people are worthy of respect and consideration, not all employees will have the skills or the desire to "fill a seat on the bus."

It is imperative that the health care team understands and commits to the practice mission and that all individuals agree to living it out on a daily basis. It is important to recognize that not all employees want to be team players. This characteristic does not make them bad people, but it may mean that they do not fit the needs of the practice. They may have great technical ability but a low level of interpersonal skills or capacity. If a leader has decided that the team model rather than the work group model is the desired aim for the health care team, this individual's lack of fit must be addressed so that the team evolution is not hampered. Although the employee may be great at a specific job or task, they are not "on the bus" and may negatively impact the team formation. It is wise to help this type of employee understand that working for the mission and the formation of the team are not optional. Not addressing this mismatch of employee ability or desire puts the entire team formation and maintenance in jeopardy, and is one of the major reasons that true teams fail to materialize.

TEAMS AND EMOTIONAL INTELLIGENCE

It must again be stressed that it is critical that practice values drive the hiring process, whereby potential employees are selected for their fit with the culture and the organizational mission. This consideration requires that employees be hired not just for their technical skills and experience but also for their interpersonal skills or emotional intelligence (EI). EI, a term and quality being used widely in the business sector, is defined as "the capacity for recognizing our own feelings and those of others, for motivating ourselves, and for managing emotions [well] in ourselves, and in our relationships" [12]. Hire for relational competency and a positive attitude. Once employees begin working, ensure that they understand that the practice and the team genuinely live out a mission and a set of values in all day-to-day interactions. A new employee quickly adapts to, and begins to emulate, the culture in which he or she works. Attracting and hiring people who exhibit team values and working to ensure that they become acquainted with the practice mission and culture early in their tenure increases the likelihood that the team attitude and aptitude will remain positive and healthy.

BUILDING TEAMS

Although teams are the preferable work unit for medical practices, they are, as previously stated, difficult to achieve. They are complex and dynamic and must be formed with care and managed with knowledge and skill. They do not just happen. Human nature is such that individuals, no matter how bright, well-trained, or committed, need a great deal of help and coaching to form a workable team.

Let us examine the most common pitfalls. There are three common assumptions made by managers and leaders that include the beliefs that their working group (1) knows how to be a cohesive team, (2) understands and accepts the value of working as a team, and (3) has the requisite self awareness, communication skills, and self-management skills necessary to collaborate well.

Leaders also presume their staff understands their expectations and goals for the practice. In most cases such assumptions are incorrect and often lethal. The first rule in leading a team is to make all things relating to the governance and expectations of the practice explicit. Just as human beings are not born knowing how to be a good marriage partner or parent, employees do not automatically have the skills or aptitudes to be true members of a team.

Moving from a traditional work group model in which individuals complete their tasks separately and independently to a team environment in which members are expected to adhere to team standards, engage in joint responsibilities, and assume accountability for practice viability and success is a major paradigm shift. The veterinary leader must make the conscious decision to create a medical team within a practice and help employees understand and commit to this new way of functioning.

CLARIFYING PURPOSE

A veterinary practice can be many things to many people. It is a place where companion animals can get excellent medical care. It can provide trustworthy diagnostic equipment and a top-of-the-line surgery suite. A practice is both an employer and a financial contributor to a community. It is a workplace and career venue for owners and associates. But what is its ultimate reason for being? Every practice owner and associate must answer this question individually and corporately.

Most veterinarians, if they were to ponder this question, would probably envision their practice as a place where all work efforts are geared toward improving the quality of life of their patients, their clients, their team, and themselves. This is a practice vision. It is bigger than the day-to-day operations and provides a clear road map for general success. This type of purpose provides a baseline against which all aspects of clinic activity can be measured.

A practice's mission or purpose needs to be clear and made explicit to the veterinary health care team. This purpose acts as the "north star" by which the practice navigates. Although the purpose is set by the leader, the specifics of what this means and how this looks in the daily operations is often set and determined by the team. People in teams expect leadership "to create the direction, alignment, and commitment that enable them, working together, to achieve organizational success" [13]. In this way, the practice owner decides the "why," but leaves it to the team to help determine the "how." This process promotes buy-in and a sense of ownership among team members. Note, too, that the mission addresses not just care of the patient and the client but also the internal practice audience, the health care team. By measuring all major (and most minor) decisions against this standard, the entire practice benefits.

PRACTICE VALUES

A mission or purpose illustrates an organization's values, or guiding principles. Established values that define what a medical entity stands for provide a clear roadmap for employees as they attempt to define their fit within the organization. Management research indicates the companies that outperform their competitors in the long run do so because they are strongly oriented toward a set of guiding values. Medical care at its best is values driven. Characteristics such as warmth, empathy, expertise, insight, communication, and extraordinary effort permeate practices that receive high marks from patients, clients, and employees alike. "When team relationships work well and morale is high, it is often because team members share similar values and these in turn are invariably modeled right from the top of the organization—through the leadership" [14].

Strong values, a compelling mission, attention to the work-life climate and the satisfaction of a team have proven power in the establishment of a successful organization. Shared values and a common purpose create a sense of team identity, which is an integral component of successful teams.

FOCUS ON RELATIONSHIP

At the organizational level, a positive climate is reinforced through support of appropriate employee behaviors and concern for their well-being [15]. The focus of a values-driven, mission-based organization is on relationships and technical competencies. Employees must hear this message loud and clear. The quality of their relationships with one another and with clients is as important as their technical expertise and work. Until this idea permeates the work culture, true teamwork will not occur.

Some leaders, however, balk at this concept and do not believe it is their role to encourage or enforce employees' positive behavior with team members. This belief, more than any other, inhibits team development and allows work groups to perpetuate dysfunctional work behaviors. It is the leader's responsibility to establish and reinforce a positive team culture.

This new culture may be arduous to enforce, but it is worth the effort. Changing habituated behavioral patterns is challenging, but with persistence it can be done. The payoff is great. Once a team begins to see the benefits of an improved work climate, they themselves will take on its reinforcement. This phenomenon occurs because attention to workplace values and team building promotes a human need for connection, for belonging, and for being a part of something greater than the individual. Most people, given the opportunity, would choose to work in a place that respects their need for collegiality and values their contributions. As employees are hired and acclimated to fit this new, more productive team model, relationship management becomes much less time intensive as it becomes the normal office climate.

TEAM INGREDIENTS

We have clarified the difference between a work group and a team and have made the case for health care teams to be actual teams in every sense of the word. We will now investigate how to implement many of the principles discussed into a working model for practices. In his book *The Five Dysfunctions of a Team* Lencioni [16] states that all teams must overcome potential pitfalls, which include:

- Absence of trust
- Fear of conflict
- Lack of commitment
- Avoidance of accountability
- Inattention to results

Each one of these foundational underpinnings is integral to a team's success or can contribute to a team's demise or stillbirth. Let us examine these qualities more specifically [16]. Each feature will be illustrated by a scenario example. As you read them, consider which elements are present or absent in your practice.

The Absence of Trust

Veterinary scenario

In Dr. Jones' practice, Mary has been the business manager for many years, giving her seniority over most of the other staff members. Unfortunately, Mary is not a people person. As a matter of fact, she has many prejudices and biases about people with different backgrounds and ethnicities from her own. Although good at the business end of the practice, Mary makes snide comments and jokes to certain members of the office staff. When confronted, Mary denies both her prejudices and her inappropriate behavior, and then finds subtle ways to retaliate against employees who question her. Dr. Jones depends on and supports Mary because she knows his office better than anyone and he believes he cannot afford to lose her. Although several employees have shared their distress with him regarding Mary's behavior, he always defends her and indicates he does not want to pursue these discussions.

Trust is damaged when commitments are broken, conflict is not dealt with, and destructive behavior on the part of the leader or the team is left unchecked.

In positive, productive health care teams, members have a history with one another that promotes respect and honesty. At a fundamental emotional level, employees know and accept that they are all there to promote the mission and goals of the practice, and they understand and accept one another's strengths and weaknesses. Because no team member is perfect and all team members are human, trust allows people to admit their vulnerabilities in a climate of respect and acceptance. Team members may have good and bad days without bringing down the group or creating undue conflict. Difficulties, such as negative attitudes, power struggles, or persistent competitiveness, may surface, but the foundation of trust, respect, and joint accountability provides an avenue and the safety for these issues to be addressed.

Trust such as this is built by encouraging relationship development between employees. This development does not mean everyone in the office must become friends but it does mean that they must seek to interact respectfully, assist one another in carrying out the practice mission, and understand one another's difficulties and challenges. Conflict cannot be ignored or downplayed. Employees need to understand that both they and their coworkers are held to the same standards and norms, and that breaches will be addressed.

Again, we reiterate that a group of people, no matter how motivated, does not immediately turn into a working team. True teamwork is not our normal state. People have been accustomed since childhood to seeing others as competitors for promotions or rewards and to wanting to realize their own agendas. In a longstanding work group there may be feelings of resentment or personality difficulties hindering the working relationships. To move forward, the health care team must learn to manage these problems by developing team norms to neutralize or contain these hindrances. This is where the work of teams begins.

In their recent text *The Discipline of Teams*, Katzenbach and Smith [17] list several attendant norms that they suggest the team ought to address and adopt.

- Attendance (work day and meetings)
- Appropriate interruptions (eg, when are phone calls appropriate)
- No sacred cows (no issues protected from discussion in constructive way)
- Constructive criticism (how to work through problems in a constructive way)
- Confidentiality (sensitive team issues will not be discussed outside the group)
- Action orientation (their purpose is to act and produce results)

To move employees who have been functioning as a work group toward the more effective team model, the leader needs to compare how this list of values stands against the current reality of the practice performance. Once the health care team understands the mission of the group, this next step allows them to begin to develop a culture of trust and consistency. Norms are best set by having a group meeting in which the team decides what the appropriate norms of behavior are for work relationships and what type of work climate they aim to create. Although these items are somewhat universally accepted, it is up to the team to set the norms they want to work and live by.

Some additional suggestions [8] include encouraging risk taking and creativity, outcome for handling failure or mistakes, fostering relationships and individuality, and encouraging a playful attitude. As the leader, it is important to set the tone for a norm-setting meeting by reminding the group that mutual respect, open discussion, and collaborative behavior are expected during all meetings and office interactions.

These norms set the stage for the evolution of the team's working climate. Each member of the group must participate in selecting these norms and agree to their adoption. When a new employee is hired, orientation to the team norms and climate expectations are part of the orientation to the office. This responsibility should be designated to the training employee. If this climate is upheld and modeled, new hires will quickly adapt to the acceptable modes of behavior.

The Fear of Conflict

Veterinary scenario

The Happy Tails Clinic has had constant turnover since it opened its doors 5 years ago. The two founding veterinarians, Drs. Smith and Hall, had gone to veterinary school together and have worked hard to establish a full-service clinic with a healthy work team; they do not understand why their efforts are not paying off. They put a great deal of effort into hiring people of integrity and strong work ethic and provided solid training for them. What they did not recognize, however, was that their work styles were very different. Dr. Smith believes in staying on time with appointments at all costs and has her technicians do much of the client education and returning of phone calls. Dr. Hall enjoys client contact and prefers to do all of these tasks himself, which often causes him to be behind in the schedule. His technicians often struggle with keeping him on track and this creates daily struggles with the front desk people. Both the front desk staff and Dr. Smith's technicians are frustrated with the constant discrepancy in time and work between the two vet groups and express their irritation through subtle undermining of Dr. Hall's group. No one ever brings this reality up at staff meetings because everyone knows that Dr. Smith and Dr. Hall are great friends and dislike talking about these differences.

Leaders and teams often avoid group conflict at all costs because they view it as destructive and time intensive. Such a perception is a costly miscalculation. Conflict is a normal outcome of groups of people working together. It will always exist to some degree. The key is not to do away with conflict but to manage it. Again, this takes skill and courage. People avoid conflict because they have not been taught how to work through it in a productive and professional manner.

Let us be very clear. Avoiding conflict does not mean that the underlying frustrations or discontentments disappear. Negative emotions fester and spread through a team in numerous dysfunctional ways. Organizational research and a wealth of consultant data testify to the high costs to teams, managers, and businesses resulting from the inability to effectively deal with anger and conflict in the workplace [18], including absenteeism, destructive behaviors (gossiping, subgrouping, scapegoating, and so forth), lost productivity, poor client relations, inattention to work detail, and emotional distress to all members of the team. Conflict does not go away if left unattended. It spreads and destroys the work environment and often the business environment.

Lencioni [16] describes a conflict continuum that illustrates the potential outcomes for conflict in the workplace. "On one end of the continuum there is artificial harmony with no conflict at all, and on the other there are mean-spirited, personal attacks. In the exact middle of that continuum there is a line where conflict goes from constructive to destructive or vice versa, depending on which direction the conflict goes" [16]. It seems that most organizations live closer to the harmony end of the continuum because most individuals veer away from open conflict. Lencioni recommends instead that teams work to stay near the middle of the continuum where they engage in open, constructive conflict, and air their differences or difficulties in a productive way.

This skill and the courage to engage in constructive conflict are among the most important abilities a team can master and reinforce the development of trust and faith in the team norms and values.

Conflict most often results from ineffective communication, values differences, or temperament differences. If team norms reflect the need to work through and better understand these differences, the team is freed to continue to pursue the organizational vision and mission without the deadweight of the hidden conflict.

If the team members hesitate to address conflict the practice leader or manager must do so respectfully and consistently. Team members who have identified conflicts should be asked to sit down together and practice Covey's fifth habit [1], which is to "seek first to understand and then to be understood".

CONFLICT RESOLUTION MODEL

In conflict resolution, the most important activities for all parties include verbal clarification, active listening, and accurate reflection of viewpoints and perceptions in a collegial, face-to-face discussion format. Depending on the emotional volatility of the issues or the employees, it may be necessary for a mediator or a facilitator to be present to work through these steps.

Employees who have conflicts should be encouraged to meet in a private, neutral space when they are able to do so without anger or frustration. The presence of a trusted leader or group member often helps keep emotions in check. Each employee should be given a set time (approximately 5 minutes) to summarize his or her perspective of the issue in question. During this time, the other employee takes on the role of listener or acknowledger and attempts to obtain a better understanding of the team member's perceptions through clarification and open questions. The listener then provides a brief summary of this new understanding to the others. If all agree with the conceptualization, the listener then proceeds to share his or her viewpoint, and the process is reversed.

This course of action allows the employees to stop defending their positions and to consider each other's perspective. This method, in and of itself, often results in a decrease or resolution of the conflict. At the very least, both parties have had the opportunity to be heard and understood. The mediating leader can then ask the employees to suggest solutions to the conflict based on their new understanding. If an agreement is reached, a commitment is made to try the new solution for a set period of time with the opportunity to meet and revisit the resolution at a later date to ensure compliance. If no decision is made, ground rules can be set to ensure the sanctity of the team while the employees do some reflection before meeting again. This process can be repeated as many times as is necessary to solve or mediate a conflict.

Once understanding has been achieved, team members should brainstorm a joint solution by looking for common ground. An action plan should be created and the implementation of the plan should be subject to team accountability [19].

Team members should be trained to understand that it is not conflict that gives cause for disciplinary action but the inability or refusal to deal constructively with conflict. A team culture that addresses conflict in this way will find itself freed from the destructive impact of untended conflict that plagues most workplaces.

A Lack of Commitment

Veterinary scenario

Everyone at Sunny Side Animal Clinic knows it is advertised to be "the clinic that is there when you need us." They know this because Dr. Spencer makes sure he tells every new employee that this is the clinic's mission when they start to work for him. It is even summarized on a plaque that hangs in the waiting room, where every client sees it.

Most of Dr. Spencer's employees have young children and hope to be out of the office by 5:00 PM every day. Although the office hours are on the door read "open: 7:30 AM to 5:30 PM" the staff have agreed among themselves to start turning people away at 4:45 PM. They have even locked the door early and turned the phone over to the answering service. When Dr. Spencer finally realizes what has been happening and questions his staff, they tell him that they think the mission is lofty but that their day care has to come first. They assumed he understood because he had his own children.

Lencioni [10] explains that most organizations fail to obtain commitment from their teams because they lack clarity related to the day-to-day practice application of the overall practice mission. Once a team begins to trust and respect one another and to effect successful resolution of conflict, they are ready to begin to define how their daily activities translate into the overall perpetuation of the practice's purpose for existence.

Remember, we earlier suggested a working mission might be something like "our practice is a place where all work efforts are geared toward improving the quality of life of our patients, our clients, our team, and ourselves." In adopting this type of mission, it is important to understand that no entity stays the same for long and that change is inevitable. The team should be helped to grasp that change is an ongoing process in every business and therefore must be managed. Decisions that impact the team and the practice must be discussed, not necessarily to achieve consensus but to explore individual perceptions with the goal of reaching common ground and team commitment.

The leader introduces key issues for discussion and team members are given the opportunity to react and respond. They hear each other out and they are heard. When the discussion ebbs, the leader summarizes the points made throughout the team meeting and members are given the opportunity to clarify all points to avoid misunderstandings. The leader thanks the group for their input and assures them it has been heard. The points are then taken under advisement and a decision, with full explanation of why it was made, is shared.

Team members are then asked to publicly commit to the decision and take collective ownership of its implementation. The point here is that productive team members understand that once an issue has been explored and discussed, and a decision made, it is time for the team to unite around the joint outcome. This ensures commitment to the team.

Avoidance of Accountability

Veterinary scenario

Dr. Carlson has provided colored lab coats for all employees in her office to ensure a uniform professional look among the staff. Everyone seemed excited to get the coats and agreed to wear them during clinic hours. Miranda, the lead technician, is a free spirit who makes it known that she dislikes conformity. Although she was unhappy about the office uniform concept, she was asked by Dr. Carlson to set a good example for the rest of the staff and wear it. She agreed, but now "forgets" her jacket several times a week. Dr. Carlson suspects this is her way of remaining free of the edict, but hates to confront her about it. Miranda is a whiz at her job and she does not want to chance upsetting her. She is beginning to notice other employees forgetting their jackets also. She does not say anything to the rest of the staff, because she knows they will question her lenience with Miranda.

Lencioni [10] defines accountability as "the willingness of team members to remind one another when they are not living up to the performance standards of the group." It is imperative that accountability become a norm in a productive health care team. Accountability extends beyond work or task results into the realm of team member behavior, including interpersonal behavior related to team goals, mission, and agreed-upon norms. Once a team has set its norms and defined its ideal culture, those designations become the baseline against which all work outcomes and interpersonal behavior is measured. Such indices are never meant to be seen as black and white, nor should they ever be used to validate disrespectful behavior. They merely provide guidelines and a framework that all team members understand, commit to, and strive to uphold.

Accountability must be modeled by the practice leader if it is to become an acceptable means of keeping the group on track. Achieving and maintaining a system of team accountability is a difficult accomplishment, again because people are hesitant to confront one another in even the most constructive and respectful ways. This confrontation may be more difficult on a positive team, because members will be hesitant to rock the boat and risk discord. It is imperative that the team be helped to understand that accountability is the steering mechanism that keeps the group on track, moving toward practice goals and, ultimately, the practice mission.

It is to be expected that all individuals periodically lose track of the general aim of the team. Respectful, constructive feedback about how an individual's behavior or productivity is not fulfilling the agreed-upon levels is a gift. This feedback provides the individual with the opportunity to self-reflect and make a course correction if necessary. Providing this kind of feedback as early as possible improves the chances of receptivity and success.

Inattention to Results

Veterinary scenario

At the beginning of the New Year, the Springfield Clinic held an all-staff meeting to let employees know about the plan to build a new clinic the following year. The doctors urged all employees to work together to help save costs and cut expenditures wherever possible during the upcoming months to help them cover the additional expenditures expected with the new building. The entire team reacted enthusiastically and pledged to help save money. Everyone left excited about the upcoming changes.

Six months later, as the practice owners were going over the financial reports, they noticed several new expenditures for additional office equipment, an increase in laundry costs, and new shelving for pet care products for the waiting room. When questioned, the employees all had valid reasons to justify their specific expenditures and were surprised to realize that the owners were upset. Although they realized the office was committed to a cost-neutral year, none saw the harm in their small additional expenditures, which made life easier in each of their work areas.

Once a team has developed a climate of trust, reached an understanding for addressing conflict, is truly committed to team goals and norms, and is accountable to the well-being of the team, it is vital that practice outcomes and results are clarified. If the health care team's mission or vision is the ultimate destination then the acknowledged results are the milestones along the way that indicate the team is going in the correct direction and navigating by the practice's north star, its mission.

The problem with most practice results is that they are either too complex to be translated into an outcome that can be grasped or they are never monitored and shared with the group. Imagine an athlete in training who has set goals for himself but never checked to see if he was on track with achieving them. Or picture the same athlete adding to his training goals the aims of weight loss, stock market gains, and marriage to an as yet unmet bride. Obviously, there will be a great deal of stress and confusion in the mind of this young athlete as to which goals need to be addressed first. In a practice setting it is wise to set one or two simple, concrete, measurable goals and assess them each month. As these goals become achieved and incorporated into the practice culture, new goals can be introduced and set. Lencioni [16] recommends that the leader establish two goals at a time. The first should address some outgoing metrics of the team, such as client satisfaction, revenue increases, scheduling flow, and so forth. The second goal should address some element of the team's culture or climate that needs improvement.

Members should clearly understand the expected outcome of these team goals and hold one another accountable for their achievement. Results should be displayed or discussed often, so that the team has a clear picture of its accomplishments. Lencioni [16] likens this to the scoreboard at a sporting event. All members of the team always know what they are aiming for and are aware of the team results. Keeping the scoreboard, or verifiable results, prominent in the team's view keeps motivation high and reinforces team efforts.

THE CHALLENGE

With all the research data underscoring the importance of excellent team functioning to medical and veterinary health care, why is it such a rare occurrence to see medical teams trained to function in this way? The simple answers are time and money. Establishing the clarity of mission, values, and interpersonal norms outlined in this chapter would mean taking time out of busy, productive practice time or even out of staff and DVM personal time. A recent report in the *Journal of the American Medical Association* [20] states that the barrier to the development and maintenance of the primary care team is "hamster health care." This metaphor illustrates that busy medical professionals, like hamsters, are ensconced on their treadmill of urgent daily activities that eat up time that might be better spent in planning and reflection. This allegorical treadmill, on which so many medical practices run each day, is the greatest enemy to the creation of well-functioning teams. Stephen Covey [1] again provides guiding wisdom to help overcome this tedious treadmill syndrome. He urges us to put first things first and to recognize the futility of frantically running without heeding our direction or destination or making provisions for the journey. In veterinary practices, putting first things first means allocating time and money to team training and development. Weekly and monthly meetings, in which the work as laid out in this article is accomplished and all members are present and focused on the business of the team, are a wise investment for the practice.

TAKING ACTION

Few would deny the importance of true teamwork to the practice of veterinary medicine. High-functioning teams provide the potential for better, more efficient care, an improved bottom line, and an improved quality of work life for the entire staff. This means the health care team and its leader must commit to set meeting and training times in which these skills and foundational attitudes and aptitudes can be developed and supported. Although difficult to schedule and costly to hold, ongoing team meetings are essential. They provide the time and place for important conversations to take place, conflicts to be resolved, and mission course corrections made. These interludes are good preventative medicine (Appendix 1). How could veterinary practices and health care teams prescribe anything less for their own well-being?

Healthy team cultures can become a reality in even the most difficult practice environment. It means committing to making the ongoing maintenance of the team a major priority. It means hiring well. It means the practice leader persistently calls employees to function at this higher level. It means effort and perseverance on the part of everyone involved. It means a unified and united health care team. The payoff for these efforts will impact every level of the practice.

APPENDIX 1. THE VETERINARY HEALTH CARE TEAM: GOING FROM GOOD TO GREAT

Practice Exercise

Ask all employees to read this article and to use it to think through the current organizational structure of the practice. Tell them there will be a series of four meetings over the next month in which each of these elements will be discussed and explored.

First meeting
- Begin the meeting with a review of what you, as the leader, see as the strengths of your practice and your work team. Share what you see as your strengths as a veterinarian and as a leader. Share your practice vision, as you currently see it and as you would like to see it evolve.
- Invite your employees to share in the same way, stating their strengths as workers and as leaders, and how they see the current and future practice vision.
- Ask employees to list the current practice strengths and weaknesses as discussed in the article. Keep notes on all of these elements.
- Challenge them to begin to consciously watch how they interact with each other and clients and patients over the next week.

Second meeting
- Have each person share some insights about their own behavior that they discovered over the past week (each person can only describe own behaviors).
- Based on this input, have each person (veterinarians also) commit to practicing one behavior change over the next week. Take note of these behavior commitments.
- Have each person share one thing they would like to see change in the practice interpersonal climate (these should be general and not aimed at any one person). Take note.

Third meeting
- Have employees (and vets) check in with their successes and failures surrounding the new behavior practice (keep this light).
- Ask employees to provide thought and input to the following questions:
  What is the overall mission or purpose of our practice?
  What are the values we believe underpin our practice?
  Who are all of our constituencies and how do we attend to them?
  How would we like to enhance our work climate?
  Are we a work group or a team?
  If a group, how can we work at becoming more of a team? This is first outcome result to be monitored throughout the upcoming month.
- Ask for a working group that can compile the thoughts into a document that lists the proposed mission, values, constituencies, and climate.

Fourth meeting
This can be a kickoff celebration for the new structure. Sharing a meal would be a nice touch.

- Ask employees to state what they have learned about themselves and their practice throughout this month. Have them share individual goals for the upcoming month.
- Have the working group present (pass out written copies) of the culmination of thoughts and ideas.

- Have the group refine each element until all believe they can agree to its standards.
- Ask each member of the team to commit to these newly set elements verbally.
- Hang the finished results at key places around work stations so that employees are reminded of their commitments.

Ongoing meetings

At least quarterly, have an employee cover these team standards and check to see if the team believes they are being followed or if adjustments must be made. Constantly update and correct.

References

[1] Covey S. The seven habits of highly successful people. New York: Simon and Schuster; 1989.

[2] Kohn LT, Corrigan JM, Donaldson MS. In: To err is human: building a safer health system. Washington DC: National Academy Press; 2000.

[3] Coiera E, Tombs V. Communication behaviors in a hospital setting: an observational study. BMJ 1998;316:673–6.

[4] Sutcliffe KM, Lewton E, Rosenthal MM. Communication failures: an insidious contributor to medical mishaps. Acad Med 2004;79:186–94.

[5] Brown JP, Silverman JD. The current and future market for veterinarians and veterinary medical services in the United States. J Am Vet Med Assoc 1999;215:161–83.

[6] Cron WL, Slocum JV, Goodnight DB, et al. Executive summary of the Brakke management and behavior study. J Am Vet Med Assoc 2000;217:332–8.

[7] Lewis RE, Klausner JS. Non-technical competencies underlying career success as a veterinarian. J Am Vet Med Assoc 2003;222(12):1690–6.

[8] Luecke R, Polzer JT. Creating teams with an edge. Boston: Harvard Business School Press; 2004.

[9] Hackman JR. Leading teams: setting the stage for great performances. Boston: Harvard Business School Press; 2002.

[10] Lencioni P. Overcoming the five dysfunctions of a team: a field guide. San Francisco: Jossey-Bass; 2005.

[11] Collins J. Good to great: why some companies make the leap and others don't. New York: Harper Collins; 2001.

[12] Goleman D. Emotional intelligence: why it can matter more than IQ. New York: Bantam; 1997.

[13] Drath WH. Leading together: complex challenges require a new approach. Leadersh Action 2003;23(1):3–7.

[14] Pendleton D, King J. Values and leadership. BMJ 2002;325:1352–5.

[15] Bardzil R, Slaski M. Emotional intelligence: fundamental competencies for enhanced service provision. Mg Ser Qual 2003;13(2):97–104.

[16] Lencioni P. The five dysfunctions of a team: a leadership fable. San Francisco: Jossey-Bass; 2002.

[17] Katzenbach JR, Smith DK. The discipline of teams: a mindbook-workbook for delivering small group performance. New York: Wiley; 2001. p. 118.

[18] Cloke K, Goldsmith J. Understanding the culture and context of conflict: resolving conflicts at work. San Francisco: Jossey-Bass; 2001.

[19] Sharpe D, Johnson E. Managing conflict with your boss. E-book: CCL Press; 2002. p. 25–7.

[20] Grumbach K, Bodenheimer T. Can health care teams improve primary care practice? JAMA 2004;29(10):1246–51.

Vet Clin Small Anim 37 (2007) 37–47

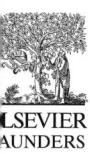

VETERINARY CLINICS
SMALL ANIMAL PRACTICE

Client-Veterinarian Communication: Skills for Client Centered Dialogue and Shared Decision Making

Karen K. Cornell, DVM, PhD[a],*, Michelle Kopcha, DVM, MS[b]

[a]Department of Small Animal Medicine and Surgery, College of Veterinary Medicine, University of Georgia, 501 South D.W. Brooks Drive, Athens, Georgia 30602-7390, USA
[b]Department of Large Animal Clinical Sciences, Practice Based Ambulatory Program, Michigan State University, East Lansing, Michigan 48824-1314, USA

"I want to be a veterinarian. I like animals and I don't want to have to deal with people." How many times have veterinarians heard this statement from individuals considering the profession of veterinary medicine? The belief that veterinarians do not need to be skilled in dealing with people, however, is a fallacy. In reality, there is a person at the "other end of the leash" (or halter) of every patient. Thus, communication is inevitable, unavoidable, and one of the most common skills employed in the day of a veterinarian. Similar to our physician counterparts, many veterinarians have traditionally believed that having and applying adequate medical knowledge to diagnose and treat patients was the only requirement for success. However, effective communication in human medicine correlates with increased career and client satisfaction as well as increased practice success [1–5]. Recent studies have confirmed the importance of communication skills within the veterinary profession and specifically identified these skills as a weakness for new veterinary graduates [6–8]. This is not surprising given that communication skills training has had minimal attention in veterinary medical curricula.

It is commonly assumed that the ability to "talk to people" or communicate effectively is an inherent attribute. In other words, "you either have it or you don't." Fortunately, studies in human medicine confirm that communication skills are not inherent and that they are just that—a set of skills that can be learned and applied effectively [9]. However, like all new techniques, for individual skills to be mastered, they must be identified, practiced, and adapted based on the outcomes they produce.

In addition to mastering the skills necessary to communicate effectively, one must also be aware of the nature of the interaction between veterinarians and their clients. Specifically, it is important to identify who holds power within the

*Corresponding author. E-mail address: kcornell@vet.uga.edu (K.K. Cornell).

0195-5616/07/$ – see front matter
doi:10.1016/j.cvsm.2006.10.005

veterinarian–client relationship. For example, is the decision-making process a shared experience or is it dominated by one party? Is the communication client-centered, doctor-centered, or relationship-centered?

Most veterinarians have established a pattern and style of communication. In many instances this style is based on a positive or negative role model they have had at some time during their career or through trial and error approaches. In this article, the authors aim to provide the practitioner with concrete descriptions of the skills that can be employed and adapted to enhance interactions with clients, colleagues, clinic staff, and others.

ROLES IN COMMUNICATION

Before discussing specific communication skills we must first explore the nature of the encounter between veterinarian and client. What is the focus of the relationship? For instance, does the veterinarian assume a dominant role and supply the client with only one option? Does the veterinarian provide only information and options with no specific recommendations? What are the communication styles or roles that are employed when interacting with clients? What are the benefits and risks associated with each of these roles?

In human medicine, three styles or roles in decision making have been described: paternalistic or guardian, consultant or teacher, and shared or collaborator [10]. Within each of these, there are four stages for interacting and information processing: acquisition of knowledge, verbal dominance, elucidation of options, and decision making [11]. The components of each of these are summarized in Table 1.

Physicians and veterinarians engage in similar interactions with their patients/clients. For example, historically, physicians and veterinarians have played the role of *guardian*. As a guardian the veterinarian is viewed as an expert who makes recommendations that the client is obliged to follow. In this type of interaction there is little discussion of what the client is capable of, desires, or requires. It is assumed that the client is comfortable with or prefers a subservient role, electing not to share decision-making power within the relationship.

The benefit of this role for the veterinarian is that clients, theoretically, will do what the veterinarian considers best. The frustration associated with the client's decision-making inabilities are minimized for both parties. An important disadvantage of this role, however, is that because decision-making power is not shared, responsibility for treatment outcomes is also not shared. In other words, if the outcome of treatment is unsatisfactory, the client will likely hold the veterinarian solely accountable.

Alternatively, the veterinarian may assume the role of *teacher*. As teacher, the veterinarian is merely a source of data and services. No opinion or recommendation is provided, leaving the client to assimilate the information and make decisions according to the data provided. Within this relationship context, decision making is entirely the responsibility of the client. The major advantage of this role for the veterinarian is that responsibility for these outcomes rests

Table 1
Roles in decision making

Stages	Guardian	Teacher	Collaborator
Acquiring knowledge	All information provided by the veterinarian	Client obtains information from the veterinarian but also from many other sources	Medical information provided by veterinarian; information relevant to preferences of client provided by client
Verbal dominance	Conversation dominated by the veterinarian	Conversation dominated by the veterinarian	Shared decision-making power; the veterinarian and client are approximately equal in the conversation
Elucidation of options	Typically only the option the veterinarian feels is best is presented	All options are presented but no weight given to veterinarian treatment preferences	All options are given; preferences of veterinarian and client are provided
Decision making	Veterinarian is the primary decision maker	Client is the primary decision maker	Shared decision making between client and veterinarian

squarely on the shoulders of the owner. A significant disadvantage of the teacher role, however, is the frustration that may result for the veterinarian when clients do not choose the "right" option. In other words, the veterinarian may have an unspoken preference for a specific treatment, but the client may choose an alternate plan. In addition, veterinarians who serve only in the capacity of teacher may find that their clients seek out multiple opinions from possibly questionable sources, thus arming the client with inaccurate information or enabling the client to delay or avoid the decision-making process entirely. This may adversely affect the health of the patient.

The third role is that of *collaborator*. Viewed by many as the optimal choice for both veterinarian and client, collaborators provide information and education regarding diagnostic and treatment options, and make explicit their professional opinions. Of equal importance, collaborators acquire information regarding client preferences, desires, and needs. The perspectives of the client are actively sought, thus allowing any barriers that may impact the diagnosis, treatment, and adherence process to be more readily identified and negotiated.

Because collaborators actively encourage client participation in decision making, a partnership in care is formed. Termed *relationship-centered care* [1], this partnership is one of shared decision-making responsibility and outcome accountability. Because clients become equal stakeholders in the decision-making process, they are more committed to codeveloping feasible strategies for treatment. Ultimately, a collaborative decision-making process may produce higher rates of client adherence to proposed treatment plans.

Literature from human medicine suggests relationship-centered interactions promote higher levels of client and physician satisfaction, improved patient health outcomes, and fewer malpractice claims [2–5]. For example, Levinson and colleagues [5] reported that significant communication differences existed between primary care physicians who had malpractice claims made against them (claims group), and those who had never had a claim made against them (no-claims group). Compared with the claims group physicians, no-claims physicians demonstrated increased numbers of statements of orientation, including the education of patients about what to expect and the flow of a visit, and greater use of facilitation techniques such as soliciting patients' opinions, checking understanding, and encouraging patients to talk.

Understandably, veterinarians have historically expressed skepticism of relationship-centered care, believing such interactions will require additional time, result in longer client visits, and slow the pace of a busy practice. In reality the no-claims physicians in the previously mentioned study did report longer office visits by a mean of 3.3 minutes. However, when you compare 3.3 minutes with the costs and time involved in defending a lawsuit, one may conclude that the initial investment of time upfront is time well spent [5].

Recently Shaw and colleagues [12] investigated veterinarian–client–patient communication patterns used during clinical appointments. In this study, two communication styles were identified—biomedical and biolifestyle. The biomedical style, reflecting a guardian approach to interaction, was identified in 58% of appointments. A relationship-centered or biolifestyle-social approach was used in 42%.

Intuitively, one might hypothesize that individual veterinarians favor a specific style of communication and therefore use it preferentially. However, results of the Shaw study indicate that the majority of veterinarians often used both styles. In fact, when evaluating the series of six videotaped client interviews for each veterinarian, 46% of veterinarians used predominately the biomedical pattern, 38% used a mixed pattern of communication (three interviews were predominately biomedical and three were predominately biolifestyle social), and 16% used a predominately biolifestyle-social pattern.

The type of appointment (eg, wellness versus medical problem) was strongly correlated with the communication pattern demonstrated. Specifically, a biolifestyle-social pattern was used in 69% of wellness appointments, whereas 85% of the medical problem appointments used the biomedical pattern.

Correlations were also identified between the style of communication and gender of individuals involved. When participants were of the same sex, communication patterns were more biolifestyle social. However, if individuals were of the opposite sex, interviews were rated as more biomedical in nature. In contrast to the study of claims versus no-claims physicians cited earlier, Shaw and colleagues reported that biomedical pattern appointments were longer in duration than those employing a biolifestyle-social pattern.

Although it is reasonable to believe that relationship-centered care is ideal, it is important to recognize that communication patterns are influenced by many factors relating to the client, the veterinarian, the nature of the visit, and the practice setting. Client-associated factors may include age, gender, and educational background. Elderly individuals may prefer a more biomedical or guardian-based relationship as these are the models to which they have grown accustomed. The nature of the visit also impacts the pattern of communication. For example, in an emergency visit, it may be more appropriate early in the encounter to employ a guardian or biomedical style of communication.

Levinson and colleagues [11] recently reported the results of a population-based study of public preferences for medical decision making in United States households. In the study, 96% of respondents preferred to be offered choices and have their opinions solicited. However, 44% said they preferred their physician be the only source of medical information and 52% preferred the physician make the final decision concerning treatment. Thus, veterinarians must actively inquire and identify the individual preferences of their clients to adapt to their specific decision-making needs.

THE 4-E MODEL FOR VETERINARIAN–CLIENT COMMUNICATION AND THE CORE COMMUNICATION SKILLS

In 1994, Keller and Carroll [13] published the 4-E model for communication between physicians and patients. This model for complete clinical care (Fig. 1) combines the necessary biomedical tasks of a patient interview with the communication steps required to achieve a successful interaction with the patient. The model proposes four communication tasks, each of which requires mastery of specific skills to achieve success. In the following paragraphs the authors have adapted this model to veterinary–client interactions.

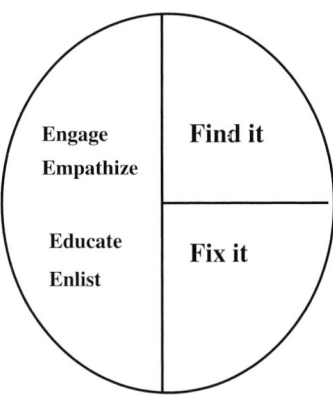

Fig. 1. Complete clinical care.

Engagement

Creating engagement is the first communication goal in a client interview. Engagement is the process of making a connection with the client to facilitate the exchange of information. To accomplish engagement the veterinarian must acknowledge and accept that each party in the interview has a unique and valuable perspective. The client is an expert regarding his/her animal and has experience and firsthand knowledge that the veterinarian does not. Although, veterinarians are experts in the areas of diagnosis and treatment of diseases, blending of both knowledge bases is required to maximize the potential effectiveness of a plan.

To make a connection, there must be an attempt by the veterinarian to form a partnership. This may be accomplished by beginning the interview with a statement of introduction and an expression of interest in the client as an individual. For example, "Good morning Mrs. Jones; my name is Dr. Smith. How are you doing today?" This personal connection puts the client at ease and facilitates the dialog and information exchange critical to attaining a diagnosis and planning appropriate therapy. The use of tangible communication skills such as open-ended questions and reflective listening techniques is recommended to facilitate the exchange of information [14].

Open-ended questions allow clients to tell their story in their own words without leading or prompting by the veterinarian. Examples of open-ended questions are provided in Box 1. Questions that incorporate "when," "what," or "where" may be helpful in eliciting relevant data. However, questions that make use of "why" should be avoided, as these types of questions could imply guilt or responsibility for the problem, and may invoke a defensive response from the client. It is important to remember that although clients will speak in response to open-ended questions, interrupting their responses may derail the course of the interview. Instead, veterinarians must focus on maintaining a calm presence with clients and using appropriate nonverbal cues such as head nodding and maintaining eye contact.

Reflective listening is a skill that uses summarizing, paraphrasing, or hypothesizing to review the information the client has shared, allowing the client to hear his/her own story as understood by the veterinarian. Reflective listening allows the client to add further information, clarify points where the story may be unclear, and correct misconceptions. Perhaps most importantly, the use of reflective listening skills communicates to the client that his/her perspective is recognized and valued, and emphasizes that they are being heard. Examples of reflective listening statements are included in Box 1.

Empathy

The second communication skill in the model outlined by Keller and Carroll [13] is empathy. Empathy is the expression of active concern for and curiosity about the emotions, values, and experiences of another [15]. Empathy suggests an appreciation for what an experience may be like for the client through seeing, hearing, and accepting the client's perspective and concerns. Examples of empathic statements are included in Box 1.

Box 1: Core communication skills and specific examples of each

Open-ended questions
Tell me about Frisky.
Tell me about what is happening with Frisky.
What happened next?
How is that going for you?
What do you think is wrong with Frisky?
Tell me more about that problem.

Reflective listening statements
It sounds like this lameness has been going on for approximately a month now and getting worse with time.
So let me see if I have this correct; the vomiting has been occurring after every meal for the last week?
You have been doing the rehabilitation exercises twice daily for three weeks; and it doesn't seem the lameness has improved?
You are concerned that because you have not seen improvement in Frisky's appetite that the treatment is not working; is that correct?

Empathic statements
You seem very concerned about Frisky today.
You look as though you are more and more frustrated with this problem.
Anyone would find this time difficult. It is so hard to go through this with a pet.

There are several methods for acknowledging the client's experience. One is a nonjudgmental response. This can be demonstrated through the use of statements such as, "This is a tough decision and there is no right or wrong answer." Another technique is normalization of the experience for the client through the use of statements like, "It is completely normal to struggle with this decision," or "Many of us are caught off guard by an emergency." The use of appropriate self-disclosure provides another option for demonstrating acceptance. Self-disclosure may include a statement such as, "I have had a pet that had cancer and it was a difficult process for me too."

Although most veterinarians acknowledge they desire empathy from their own physicians, studies suggest it is a skill many veterinarians are uncomfortable using with their clients. In fact, in a study of communication between veterinarians and clients, empathic statements were expressed in only 7% of appointments [16].

Veterinarians sometimes perceive empathy as a "soft skill" or a technique that is too "warm and fuzzy" to be applied in the context of a medical interview. Discomfort with using empathy may arise from an underlying fear that such a skill will elicit strong emotional responses from the client. Common concerns from veterinarians include, "What if I say something empathic like,

'You seem very concerned about Frisky,' and the client starts to cry? What do I do then? How am I supposed to respond?"

One way to approach these types of responses is to consider first how you would want to be treated in a similar situation. What would be the responses most appropriate for you? What preferences might others have in such a situation? In truth, people's needs vary and the best response may simply be listening without judging or feeling compelled to fill up the moments of silence that may occur.

Throughout the interview the veterinarian must attend to the client's needs and encourage client input. It is important to identify the agenda from the perspective of both individuals. It is reasonable to inquire about what the client would ultimately like to achieve during the current visit (eg, "What were you hoping we would accomplish today?"). After identifying the client's agenda, the veterinarian must provide the client with his/her own list of agenda items. It is then important that the final agenda for the visit be negotiated based on mutually decided goals and priorities that are clearly outlined. Throughout the encounter the veterinarian must provide appropriate nonverbal cues and read the nonverbal communication of the client. For more on nonverbal communication, see the article by Carson elsewhere in this issue entitled, "Nonverbal Communication in Veterinary Practice."

Education

The education portion of the interview process includes providing medical facts, opinions, and options. This includes assessing the client's perspective of the problem, providing answers to questions clients may have (whether or not they are conveyed explicitly by the client), and assuring client understanding of what has been discussed in the visit. Use of the four core communication skills, open-ended questions, reflective listening, expression of empathy and attention to nonverbal cues is critical in achieving client understanding. For example, the use of an open-ended question and an empathic statement together, such as, "How are you doing with the information I have provided so far? I know this is a lot of information to absorb in a very short time" invites the client to ask additional questions and gain further understanding.

Reflective listening on the part of the client may also be encouraged so that the veterinarian may accurately assess client understanding. This type of interaction might be a statement such as, "I know you are not the only person who cares for Frisky. It is a challenge to understand all that we have gone over today and it can be even more difficult to explain it to someone else. Would you like to tell me what you are going to tell your partner about this? Then I can address any questions that might arise."

This series of statements and questions includes the use of empathy and encourages the client to reflect their understanding of what has transpired during the visit. It is crucial to pay close attention to nonverbal messages during this type of encounter. First, the veterinarian's nonverbal message must be congruent. For example, a demeaning tone of voice with the statements used previously might create an unsafe environment for the client to share his/her understanding of the content discussed. Reading the client's nonverbal cues for understanding is also helpful. The client who shakes her head no and furrows her brow, while verbalizing, "yes I can provide the necessary treatment," is sending a mixed message. This is a cue that she is not confident in her ability to provide care. It is also important that veterinarians provide information in the language of the client. This means adapting the medical jargon of every day veterinary medical conversation into terms that can be understood by someone who is not trained in a medical profession. Although abbreviations such as *CBC, UA, DJD, VD,* and *BAR* are commonplace for veterinarians, they may not be readily understood by a majority of clients.

Enlistment

The procedure of enlistment includes two processes: decision-making and encouraging adherence [13]. The goal of these is to encourage client responsibility in making decisions and implementing treatment. In the decision-making process it is important to investigate the client's beliefs and convictions. Does he have confidence in the accuracy of his pet's diagnosis?

Client "buy-in" to the diagnosis promotes greater success in treatment adherence and treatment outcomes. For example, the client who does not believe her cat's inappropriate urination is due to behavioral issues but rather due to infection will be dissatisfied with anything less than treatment with antibiotics. If the veterinarian does not make the effort to explore the client's perspective, the result may be a disgruntled client, a frustrated veterinarian because the recommended plan was not implemented, and a cat that is still urinating inappropriately!

To achieve adherence the veterinarian must also assure there is client understanding. For example, in the case of a dog that has a urinary tract infection, the client must understand the importance of completing the full course of antibiotic therapy to avoid placing her pet at unnecessary risk of recurrent and resistant infection. Steps the veterinarian may take to help increase the likelihood of client adherence include: keeping the regimen simple, writing the regimen out in clear and simple terms, providing pictures if necessary, motivating the client by giving specific information about the benefits of treatment and the risks of not treating or treating inappropriately, preparing the client for side-effects, thoroughly discussing any obstacles they perceive regarding the mutually agreed upon plan, and finally, asking the client for their input and evaluating their conviction to the plan.

In summary, veterinarians who wish to improve their communication with clients must first understand that there is no perfect model. Each client must be viewed as an individual with specific needs. It is the responsibility of the veterinarian, with the aid of the core communication skills we have discussed, to identify and adapt to each client's needs. Studies in the human medical literature support the concept that a majority of patients wish to have a relationship-based interaction and that this type of interaction may be facilitated by use of the 4-E model of communication (Appendix 1).

APPENDIX 1

Mastery of the communication skills discussed within this article requires practice and feedback. The following exercises are designed to allow integration and repeated practice of core communication skills in a low-risk setting, with feedback provided by fellow participants. Prior to beginning these exercises it is recommended that participants review Table 1 and Box 1.

EXERCISE 1

In this exercise, participants should be divided into groups of three. Participant A will be the interviewer, participant B will be the interviewee, and participant C will be the observer. The objective of this exercise is to incorporate the core communication skills—open-ended questions, reflective listening, and expression of empathy—into a nonwork-related conversation. Before beginning the interview, the interviewer should outline two or three specific goals for the interview. Examples of specific goals include, "I want to use two open-ended questions" or "I will employ one empathic statement during this interview." This interview should take approximately 5 minutes followed immediately by 3 to 5 minutes of feedback.

Participant A

1. Set two goals for incorporating core communication skills into the interview process.
2. Interview participant B regarding his/her most recent visit to the dentist (or other health care provider).

Participant B

1. Respond to questions asked of you by participant A.

Participant C

1. Listen carefully to the interaction between participants A and B. Provide concrete and specific feedback to participant A related to the goals that were agreed upon before the exercise.
2. Write down specific examples in quotes. For example you might say, "you used two-open ended questions including, "Tell me a little bit about..." and, "Tell me more..." It is important that specifics be identified. Avoid generalized descriptive feedback such as, "That was good."

EXERCISE 2

In this exercise, the three participants from the previous exercise will rotate roles and now conduct/observe an interview within a veterinary clinic examination room. Participant A will be the interviewer amd should perform the role they actually fulfill in their real work environment. For instance, if participant A is a veterinarian, he/she will play the part of a veterinarian. If participant A is a veterinary technician or a veterinary receptionist, he/she should conduct the interview in the role of a veterinary technician or receptionist (eg, the receptionist would greet the client and interact with the client just as he/she would in a real work environment).

Participant B is the client and has come into the clinic today to have his/her dog Killer examined for lameness.

Participant C is the observer.

As in Exercise 1, the interviewer should establish goals in advance and the observer should provide specific feedback. This exercise may be repeated with each participant rotating through each of the roles. Be sure to have participants function within their real life role so that the experience is as realistic as possible and the results of this exercise may be directly applied to the work environment. The exercise may be increased in difficulty, by having the client be more or less responsive, or angry, or difficult. Take care that participants are comfortable with the process before increasing the difficulty of the interview.

References

[1] Roter DL, Stewart M, Putnam SM, et al. Communication patterns of primary care physicians. JAMA 1997;277:350–6.

[2] Hall JA, Dornan MC. Meta-analyses of satisfaction with medial care: description of research domain and analysis of overall satisfaction levels. Soc Sci Med 1988;27:637–44.

[3] Stewart MA. Effective physician-patient communication and health outcomes: a review. Can Med Assoc J 1995;152:1423–33.

[4] Levinson W. Physician-patient communication. A key to malpractice prevention. JAMA 1994;272:1619–20.

[5] Levinson W, Roter DL, Mullooly JP, et al. Physician-patient communication. The relationship with malpractice claims among primary care physicians and surgeons. JAMA 1997;277:553–9.

[6] Brown JP, Silverman JD. The current and future market for veterinarians and veterinary medical services in the United States. J Am Vet Med Assoc 1999;215:161–83.

[7] Cron WL, Slocum JV Jr, Goodnight DB, et al. Executive summary of the Brakke management and behavior study. J Am Vet Med Assoc 2000;217:332–8.

[8] Lewis RE, Klausner JS. Nontechnical competencies underlying career success as a veterinarian. J Am Vet Med Assoc 2003;222:1690–6.

[9] Hobma S, Ram P, Muijtens A, et al. Effective improvement of doctor-patient communication: a randomised controlled trial. Br J Gen Pract 2006;56:580–6.

[10] Charles C, Gafni A, Whelan T. Decision-making in the physician-patient encounter: revisiting the shared treatment decision-making model. Soc Sci Med 1999;49:651–61.

[11] Levinson W, Kao A, Kuby A, et al. Not all patients want to participate in decision making. A national study of public preferences. J Gen Intern Med 2005;20:531–5.

[12] Shaw JR, Bonnett BN, Adams CL, et al. Veterinarian-client-patient communication patterns used during clinical appointments in companion animal practice. J Am Vet Med Assoc 2006;228:714–21.

[13] Keller VF, Carroll JG. A new model for physician-patient communication. Patient Educ Couns 1994;23:131–40.

[14] Bonvicini K. Bayer Animal Health Communication Project. Getting the story: understanding client and patient. New Haven (CT): Institute for Healthcare Communication; 2003.

[15] Sprio H, Curnen M, Peschel E, et al, editors. Empathy and the practice of medicine. New Haven (CT): Yale University Press; 1993.

[16] Shaw JR, Adams CL, Bonnett BN, et al. A description of veterinarian-client-patient communication using the Roter Method of Interaction Analysis. J Am Vet Med Assoc 2004;225:222–9.

Vet Clin Small Anim 37 (2007) 49–63

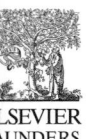

VETERINARY CLINICS
SMALL ANIMAL PRACTICE

Nonverbal Communication in Veterinary Practice

Cecile A. Carson, MD*

University of Rochester Medical Center, 7982 Williams Road, Honeoye, NY 14471, USA

Clinical experience shows that until people are allowed to express their emotions, they are usually not ready to take steps toward solving their problem. Therefore, before veterinarians can help their clients to solve their animals' medical problems, they need to know how to attend to client emotions [1]. The nonverbal channel of communication is the primary form in which emotions and the meaning of a verbal communication are expressed.

When the deep feelings that people have about their pets are trivialized or ignored or when client relations issues like complaints, anger, or grief are not acknowledged with sincerity and respect, many pet owners become dissatisfied, disillusioned, and even hostile [2]. Most veterinarians are well meaning in their concern for animal health and clients, but many may not be aware of how their nonverbal behavior is affecting a vulnerable client whose feelings about his or her animal are always involved to varying degrees in a visit to the clinic. We all respond to the nonverbal behavior of others but are not often conscious of our response, and therefore lack an awareness of how to respond differently or more effectively. Fortunately, observing and responding to nonverbal behavior can be learned as a set of skills, which can be practiced and added to the veterinarian's repertoire of clinical resources.

Nonverbal communication refers to those behaviors between veterinarians and clients that reflect the tenor of how a particular interaction is proceeding. This article focuses on the nonverbal behavior between the veterinarian and the client rather than on the nonverbal aspects of communicating with and handling the animals. Nonverbal communication includes all behavioral signals that go on between interacting individuals, exclusive of verbal content, and also includes the space and environment in which the communication takes place; thus, we are communicating at all times, even if we are silent. Attention to these signals allows the veterinarian to monitor the process of an interaction, keeping a finger on the pulse of what is transpiring in a moment-to-moment

This work was originally developed through grant 72/87A from the National Fund for Medical Education.

*Williams Road, Honeoye, NY 14471. *E-mail address:* ccarson4@aol.com manner, and therefore being more able to guide the interaction in a positive direction.

Roughly 80% of all communication between individuals is nonverbal and is generally involuntary. This means that important information that cannot be hidden is being exchanged at all times—from client to veterinarian and from veterinarian to client. Twenty percent is verbal and voluntary, and therefore represents only a small proportion over which we have conscious control. This 20% is the verbal channel through which clinicians impart necessary medical information, but the remaining 80% encodes the meaning of the information to the client by bridging the gap between what is said and what is interpreted. Any problems a client is having with adherence or motivation in the animal's care is signaled in the nonverbal channel, regardless of whether or not he or she agrees verbally with the veterinarian. Conversely, any problems the veterinarian is having with the client are signaled nonverbally as well.

Attending to the nonverbal channel does not add extra time because it occurs simultaneously with the verbal interchange and is simply a process of noticing and responding as the flow of the interaction proceeds. In fact, Ambady and colleagues [3] were able to show that people are fairly accurate at identifying emotions from exposure to nonverbal behavior of only 375 milliseconds. This rapid assessment of the nonverbal message provides the veterinarian with a method for tracking how a client is feeling at any given moment and allows the veterinarian to respond in an appropriate manner. Although this is useful in all encounters with clients, it is particularly important when difficult decisions are involved, such as euthanasia and considering costly procedures.

Although most of the research in nonverbal behavior has been done in human medicine, much of it can be extrapolated into veterinary practice because it involves human-to-human interaction around a health care issue. Patient complaints in human medicine are usually a result of communication problems rather than technical competency or quality-of-care issues. In fact, a breakdown in communication and resultant patient dissatisfaction has been shown to be the most common reason underlying a complaint or malpractice claim [4]. In 1980, DiMatteo and coworkers [5] tested 71 internal medicine residents on a standard Profile of Nonverbal Sensitivity (PONS). They were able to demonstrate a positive correlation of residents' higher scores on the PONS with the measures of satisfaction in their doctors of 500 of their patients.

A large amount of nonverbal information is exchanged at all times, and it is helpful to organize this information into meaningful form to work more effectively with clients. Nonverbal data can be organized into four general categories: kinesics, proxemics, paralanguage, and autonomic shifts. Kinesics refers to such behaviors as facial expressions, general level of tension in the body, gestures, touch, and body position and movement. Most people think of this category when they hear the word "nonverbal." Proxemics refers to how the space is shaped between the client, animal, and veterinarian: vertical height differences; interpersonal distance; angles of facing; and physical barriers, such as charts, examination tables, and even the animal itself [6,7]. Spatial behavior modulates the expression of power, territoriality, protection, and alliance in an encounter. Paralanguage is the "music" of language–those nonword phenomena, such as pause, pitch, rate, intonation, volume and emphasis, that tell us so much of what someone wants to say [8]. A warm and inviting voice can create relaxation and comfort in a client and help him or her be able to more readily speak about primary concerns as well as helping the client to be more receptive when the veterinarian is in an educating mode.

If using appropriate words to describe a situation while speaking extremely fast, the veterinarian may be seen as rushed, nervous, insensitive, or unsure of himself or herself. If one speaks the same words too slowly, he or she may be viewed as dull, boring, or even condescending. It is especially important to control voice tone and pacing when working with clients who are anxious, angry, grieving, or upset. Words that are spoken softly and at a slightly slower pace than normal are viewed as more soothing and comforting [2].

The fourth category, autonomic shifts, is governed by the autonomic nervous system, and therefore is the one category over which we have little or no control. Facial color can shift from neutral to flushed or blanched, the conjunctivae of the eye can begin to glisten as an early sign of tearing, palms may become sweaty, and breathing may shift to higher in the chest versus deeper in the belly, or individuals may sometimes hold their breath in relation to a particular topic the veterinarian may have brought up. When an autonomic shift occurs, it often indicates that a person is experiencing strong feelings.

BASIC BEHAVIOR

These four categories of nonverbal behavior are useful in quickly identifying whether or not the client is feeling safe in the encounter. Safety is a basic human need involving self-protection and self-preservation, and clients need to know if the veterinarian is safe enough for them to expose their concerns, fears, and vulnerability. Clients are less receptive to their veterinarian's attempts to educate or to come to a decision about the animal's care without it.

If the client does not feel safe, he or she typically responds with the "not-safe" behaviors of fight or flight. By recognizing nonverbal input from clients in the four categories of kinesics, proxemics, paralanguage, and autonomic shifts, the veterinarian can immediately read patterns of behaviors to determine this (Table 1).

Feelings of safety are reflected by body signals of engagement, relaxation, and a physically open stance. These include little general body tension, with arms and legs relaxed and uncrossed and relaxation of facial muscles. The client who feels safe shows more variety in gestures and voice because the sense of safety gives rise to freer expression of concerns and feelings.

The stance of the client who is feeling the fight response is one of increased body tension and engagement in "attack mode" as a defense to feeling unsafe. Typical nonverbal signals of this are a forward lean with jutting jaw, clenched fists, and narrowing of the eyes with the inner brows lowered and the mouth tense. The client may also show facial flushing, nostrils flaring, hands on hips, increased voice volume, and deeper breathing.

Table 1
Nonverbal communication: basic behavior

Nonverbal category	Safety	Fight	Flight
Body and face			
Body angulation	Engaged	Engaged	Disengaged
Arms and legs	Uncrossed (open)	Fist/jaw clenched	Crossed (closed)
Body tension	Relaxed	Tensed	Tensed
Head position	Neutral (forward)	Head lowered	Turned away
Facial muscle	Face and brows relaxed	Brows furrowed, eyes narrowed	Eyes widened
Physiology			
Skin color	Neutral color	Flushed	Blanched
Breathing	Neutral or deeper in chest	Deeper in chest, increased rate	Shallow or holding breath
Voice			
Volume	Neutral/increased	Increased	Decreased
Quality	Melodious	Staccato	Strained, hesitant
Space			
Horizontal distance	Decreased	Decreased	Increased
Barriers	Down	Down	Up

Flight is also characterized by the client's increased body tension but with disengagement and withdrawal instead: leaning away, pushing or stepping back, a diminishing volume of the voice, increased rate of the breathing as it becomes more shallow or is held, and blanching of facial color. Other typical cues of the feeling of flight include putting up physical barriers (eg, crossed arms and legs), averting the eyes or turning the head away, and holding on more tightly to the animal.

It is important to read the overall pattern of nonverbal responses rather than to rely on any one sign. Clients sometimes cross their arms and legs because it is cold, because there are no arms to the chair, or as a convention of etiquette; however, their body may be quite relaxed and engaged and their voice melodious, indicating an overall sense of safety in the encounter. The degree of body tension seems to be a major indicator of safe versus not-safe, and the rest of the nonverbal signals in Table 1 can be added on from there. Mixed responses, such as fight and flight, are also frequent, especially when clients are angry but afraid to jeopardize the relationship with the veterinarian by saying so. In this instance, the client may demonstrate a flushed face and loud voice combined with crossing the arms or turning away [9].

NONVERBAL SKILLS
Helping clients move from not-safe to safe is crucial to the process of creating a therapeutic milieu in which to gather high-quality information from the client and to relax the client and the animal. "Even more than this [in the sense of safety and relaxation], the veterinarian is allowed to witness the caring of the owner as he or she shares their heart with the animal—and that gets exchanged

with the veterinarian, too, and nurtures their experience. The result of this is that there is a human to human interaction between the client and the veterinarian, with the animal acting as a catalyst, that is enriching to both parties" (S. Clark, DVM, personal communication, 2004). There are three nonverbal skills that can be used to create safety when the client is feeling not-safe.

Addressing Mixed Messages

> Beware of the man whose belly does not shake when he laughs. (Chinese proverb)

When there is incongruence between verbal and nonverbal modes in your client's communication, the nonverbal message more truly reflects the person's actual feelings and predicts his behavior in response to the negotiation at hand. The veterinarian may see a nonverbal "no" message from the client through a furrowed brow, slight shaking of the head, a strained voice, breath holding, an increase or decrease in facial color, or a tensing of the muscles. It is important to recognize that when a nonverbal "no" is offered, even if the client has agreed verbally, the veterinarian's task in communicating is not finished. If incongruence is left unaddressed, the client does not adhere to what he or she has agreed to do or has difficulty or is frustrated in attempting to do it.

A client's mixed message may be attributed to a number of factors, including but not limited to feeling that disagreeing with or questioning the veterinarian may affect the animal's care, fear or concern about new medications or regimens for the animal that may be perceived as unwarranted, concern about the expense of what is being recommended, and feeling overwhelmed or distressed.

There are two major strategies for addressing mixed messages from clients, and they both recognize that incongruence reflects the client's inability to express his or her feelings directly. Both strategies help to convert an incongruent "yes" into a congruent "no" so that the objection is openly available for discussion and collaboration. The first strategy is direct acknowledgment, which openly acknowledges that the veterinarian is receiving two messages from the client: "You know, even though you say you'll go ahead with the heartworm medicine 12 months of the year, I sense you have some hesitation about it. If you have some concerns, let's talk about them." If the client relaxes and or nods in agreement, the congruent "no" is now out on the table and the client can safely discuss it.

If, instead, the client withdraws or tenses, the second strategy may be more useful. Using the language of the "third person" avoids direct reflection to the client. Instead, it raises potential questions or fears through linguistic distancing to increase the client's feeling of safety through "saving face." The veterinarian can say, "I hear a lot of clients express concerns about giving their dog heartworm medication year round." Here, the veterinarian would look carefully at the client to see if the nonverbal parameters of agreement were present, such as head nodding, deeper breathing, return of facial color, and muscle relaxation. If the client nonverbally remains silent, the veterinarian can pursue the client's potential concerns further through the linguistic third person by saying, "One of their concerns is often about possible side effects to the dog" (again, the veterinarian would watch for nonverbal signs of agreement or disagreement) "and another one is about any additional cost." By this time, the client usually feels a clear invitation to explore any of these concerns or to offer additional ones.

This is a key skill for shared decision making of the routine but frequently difficult choices that clients and veterinarians have to make, including decisions regarding ovariohysterectomy, surgery, euthanasia, or chemotherapy. To get the client's perspective fully and freely, the two strategies can be combined with a verbal empathic statement as well, such as: "It's so hard sometimes to know what's best, isn't it?" When the veterinarian clearly indicates support regardless of the client's preference, it significantly eases the difficulty of making a decision.

Remember, too, that veterinarians send mixed messages, and when they do so, they can deliver a powerful message of not being completely trustworthy and actually make the encounter more unsafe. For example, if the veterinarian seems to be in a hurry to obtain client consent regarding a surgical procedure that the client is hesitant to pursue, the client may feel that the veterinarian is not revealing all the possible complications and may feel pushed into making a decision.

Shaping Space

How the veterinarian arranges and uses the physical space frequently parallels how he or she views the interpersonal relationship with the client. Intentionally shaping the physical space of an encounter can set the structure for reflective listening and for improving the quality of the interaction. Specific components of the space include (1) setting the stage, which relates to inviting or welcoming the client and animal into the physical space; (2) interpersonal distance, which relates to territoriality; (3) vertical height differences, which relate to power in an encounter; (4) angles of facing, which relate to alliance or partnership in the relationship; and (5) physical barriers, which relate to protection.

In setting the stage, attention is given to the nonverbal message of welcome, including physical aspects of the practice, such as adequate parking, ease of access to the building, use of a separate entrance for animals that are difficult to manage, and use of a separate exit for clients who have had their animals euthanized (to avoid other clients waiting with their [alive] companions). The waiting area may be set up to be comfortable and well lit with enough room to keep animals at a reasonable distance from each other. In addition, the waiting room space can be used to showcase framed poems or posters that refer to the joy and sadness of animal ownership and death; in addition, pictures, plaques, or artwork that memorializes special pets can be displayed [10]. A message of courtesy and convenience can also be sent through a bulletin board listing of staff names and roles to help orient new clients to the practice. By the time clients and pets reach the examination room, they have received a significant number of nonverbal messages, including those interactions with members of the front office health care team, before they encounter the veterinarian. In the examination room, consideration can be given for the client to sit or stand comfortably during the consultation and examination of the animal.

A second way to work with spatial relationships is through interpersonal distance. If the veterinarian is too close during an interview, the client feels that his or her space has been encroached on and is likely to behave in ways intended to restore proper distance. This may include looking or turning away or placing or clutching the animal between them. Alternately, being too far away discourages true engagement and may convey a sense of veterinarian disinterest in the client.

Vertical height difference is the third element of shaping space. At the start of an encounter, many clients may feel less powerful and more vulnerable relative to the veterinarian because they are dependent on his or her expertise in their concern for their animal. The veterinarian can minimize this feeling in the client by being willing to be at the same level or below whenever possible. In Fig. 1, the veterinarian is standing over the client, putting her full attention on the animal, and not noticing how this literally backs the client into a corner. The client, meanwhile, is using the dog partially as a barrier to the nonverbal experience of feeling overpowered and encroached on. In Fig. 2, the veterinarian has noticed what she is communicating nonverbally and has responded differently. Even though there is no other chair to sit on in the examination room, she has changed the height of her body by leaning against the examination table. This also causes her to move back a bit and allows the client more interpersonal distance to be able to express her concerns more easily. This seems to have helped the dog engage as well. In Fig. 3, the veterinarian is with a client couple, educating them about the anatomy of their limping animal's hip. The couple is obviously engaged in receiving the information; however, nonverbally, the relationship is more hierarchic than collaborative because of the

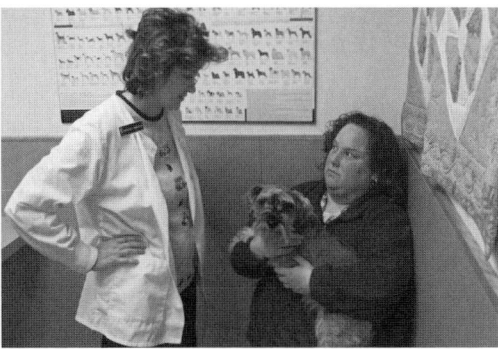

Fig. 1. Overpowering the client with vertical height difference and close interpersonal distance. (Courtesy of Bayer Animal Health Communication Project, New Haven, CT.)

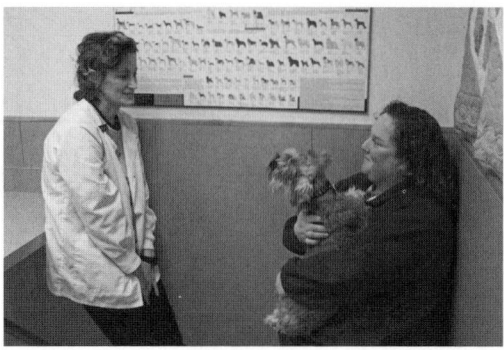

Fig. 2. Relieving vertical height difference and interpersonal crowding. (Courtesy of Bayer Animal Health Communication Project, New Haven, CT.)

height differences, and this position tends to discourage the clients from asking questions or voicing concerns. In Fig. 4, the veterinarian has been willing to go beyond "eye to eye" with her clients, sitting on the floor, which more fully invites their questions and concerns. This position also invites everyone, including the animal, to relax and feel more open.

The fourth component of shaping space is angles of facing. When the veterinarian and client disagree and are facing directly opposite each other, their physical position can cause them to experience differences as more confrontational than is actually intended. A verbal cue in this instance may include the client saying, "Yes, but. . ." Once the veterinarian is aware that a difference of opinion may exist, he or she can begin to defuse the intensity of the difference by slowly changing the angle at which he or she is facing. Just a slight angulation can begin to ease the tension. If the veterinarian moves even further into a side-by-side position with the client, the configuration more clearly supports a collaborative effort between them in spite of the disagreement. The animal

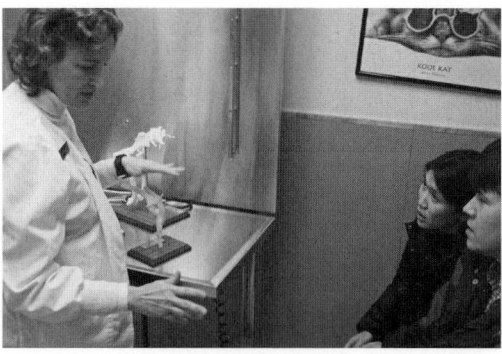

Fig. 3. Vertical height difference in educating clients: hierarchic relationship. (Courtesy of Bayer Animal Health Communication Project, New Haven, CT.)

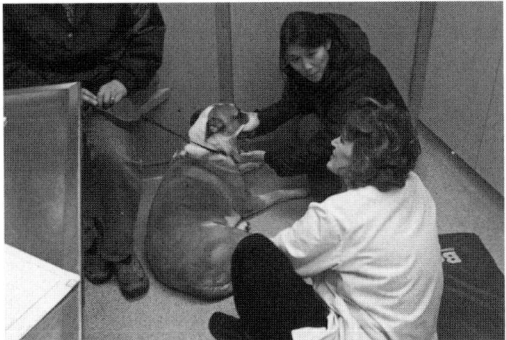

Fig. 4. Vertical height difference in educating clients: collaborative relationship. (Courtesy of Bayer Animal Health Communication Project, New Haven, CT.)

can also serve to modulate this experience if placed between the two people during this encounter: the animal's presence can diminish the confrontational aspects by serving as a barrier to the direct frontal experience of the other person. Furthermore, if both people are touching the animal, there is a message sent of connection between the people through the medium of the animal. In Fig. 5, the veterinarian has engaged her client in a position of alliance, and the client is freer to express her feelings of sadness more openly. In Fig. 6, as the veterinarian moves into a position of even greater collaboration while sharing information on the animal's record, the client begins to relax and become more connected to the material the veterinarian is trying to explain.

Physical barriers are a final component of proxemics and often send a message of "keep your distance," whether the message is intended or not. The barriers can be a reception desk, crossed arms or legs, an examination table, a chart, a crate, restraints, or, sometimes, the animal itself. In recent years, the introduction of the computer in the examination room serves as an

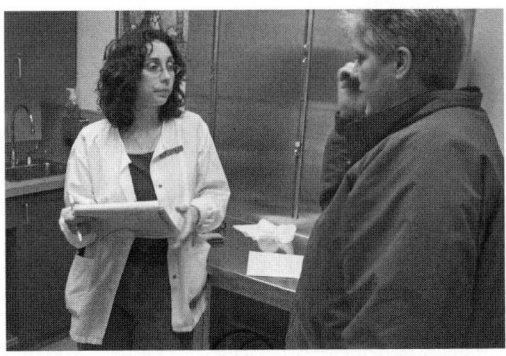

Fig. 5. Angles of facing: assisting expression of client affect. (Courtesy of Bayer Animal Health Communication Project, New Haven, CT.)

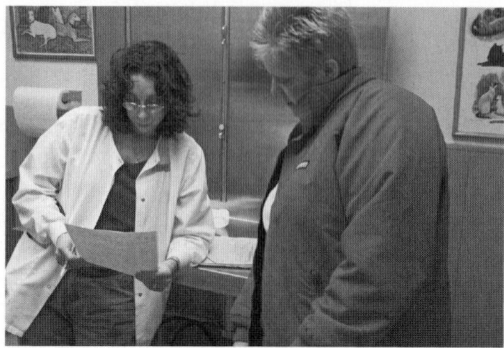

Fig. 6. Angles of facing: full collaborative position. (Courtesy of Bayer Animal Health Communication Project, New Haven, CT.)

additional barrier. Fig. 7 illustrates how an animal located between the veterinarian and the client can also be an asset as well as a barrier, because the veterinarian's contact with the cat becomes a way of connecting and making contact with the client. Fig. 8 shows the potential challenge of examination room computers as the veterinarian inadvertently turns her back to the client while concentrating on the keyboard and screen. In Fig. 9, the veterinarian has chosen to adjust the screen and keyboard to maintain more eye contact and include the client in the deliberations. She might also have chosen to retain the original position of the computer and to look over her shoulder from time to time as another way to include the client.

Developing Nonverbal Rapport

> Rapport is *the process of moving as another person moves.* Also known as interpersonal synchrony, its basic message is *"I am with you"* [11].

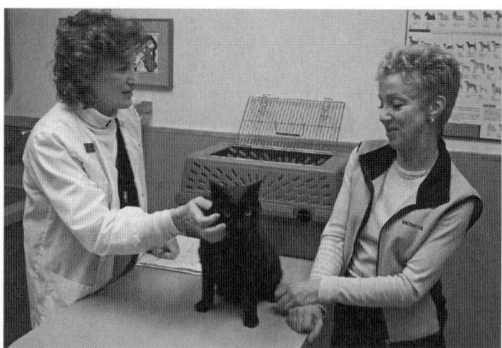

Fig. 7. Physical barriers. The animal can facilitate the connection between the veterinarian and client at times rather than being a barrier. (Courtesy of Bayer Animal Health Communication Project, New Haven, CT.)

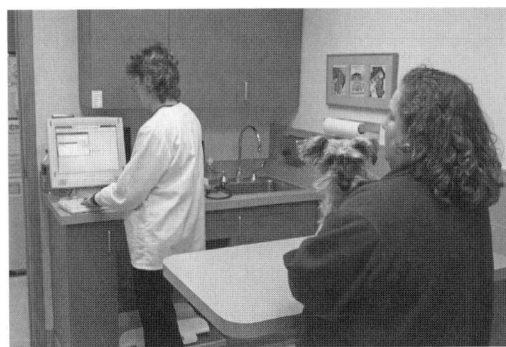

Fig. 8. Physical barriers: the computer creates a cutoff between the veterinarian and client. (Courtesy of Bayer Animal Health Communication Project, New Haven, CT.)

This moving together of veterinarian and client can be seen visually, can be heard in terms of matched voice tones or phrasing, and can be felt directly in the body by assuming postures or gestures similar to those of the other person. When the veterinarian creates this rhythm and connection with a client, he or she quite literally enters their world nonverbally and can begin to sense what the client's experience might be like. From this, a natural sense of empathy emerges. Clients recognize this nonverbal acknowledgment of their world by the veterinarian, typically through a feeling of being "understood."

Learning to recognize and create rapport is perhaps the most fundamental nonverbal skill. It creates common ground on which to build support in the relationship with the client, allowing the client to offer spontaneously all the information and associations that may be important to his or her reason for seeking help for a pet. Through such support, the client is also more likely to be receptive to the therapeutic options that are offered. Thus, it paves the way for meaningful interaction and the acquisition of high-quality information.

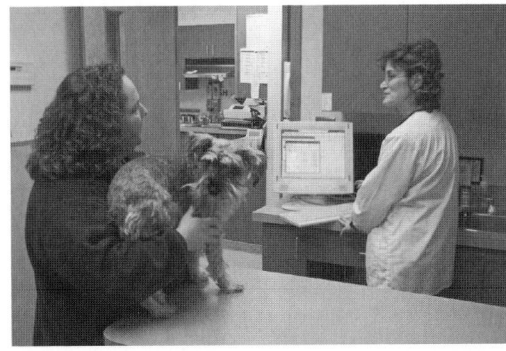

Fig. 9. Physical barriers: the computer as a tool for collaboration. (Courtesy of Bayer Animal Health Communication Project, New Haven, CT.)

There are two parts to developing nonverbal rapport: matching and leading. Matching is the process of moving as the client moves in such a way so as to acknowledge aspects of the client's behavior as a reflection of the state he or she is in. The veterinarian can match anything he or she may notice: facial expression, voice volume and rate, or body posture and gestures. For example, a guarded client who is putting up barriers of arms or an animal is likely to respond more favorably to a clinician who is in a more "closed" posture rather than a clinician who has arms open and is closing in on the interpersonal distance between them. Also, it is extremely important to be graceful and respectful in the matching and to match only enough so that what the veterinarian is doing does not come into the conscious awareness of the client; otherwise, the client feels mimicked rather than supported.

Leading is the use of the interpersonal synchrony that has been set up by matching. It is analogous to a dance, where a change of direction is easier to follow when the pair of dancers is in step. People in rapport are motivated to try to stay that way, and a leading motion by one person of a pair is quite likely to produce a reciprocal response in the other. Leading invites the client to move with the veterinarian in his recommendations or concerns rather than feeling rushed or coerced into them. If the veterinarian leads too fast or too dramatically, however, rapport may be interrupted, but it can be recovered by returning to matching. For instance, the veterinarian and client may be in synchrony in their rate of speech and in the veterinarian's mirroring the client's facial expression as the client begins to express important feelings. If in the middle of the expression of those feelings, the veterinarian reaches for the animal or the medical record and turns his or her focus toward it, however, he or she has disrupted the interactional synchrony, and the client may feel a distinct disconnection and a sense of being unsupported. This disconnection can be readily repaired by the clinician's return to the nonverbal matching once again. Additionally, any new or unexpected verbal content introduced into the interaction can also be considered "leading" from the client or from the veterinarian; for example, giving a diagnosis or recommending medications or procedures the client was not expecting are "leads," and it helps to be in interpersonal synchrony with the client when they are introduced. Conversely, if a client suggests unnecessary treatment or procedures, it is easier for the veterinarian to understand the perspective of the client's world in which that behavior makes sense by going back to nonverbal matching.

Obviously, getting into nonverbal rapport with a diversity of clients requires flexibility on the veterinarian's part, but the benefit in improved communication and client satisfaction is well worth the effort. There are some behaviors of clients that are more difficult to match. One example is raising one's voice volume with an angry client, but not one's voice tone, because it may be useful in allowing the client to recognize that his or her strong feelings are being acknowledged. Paradoxically, this often unconsciously allows the client to lower the volume and angry tone of his or her voice much more quickly. A cheerful outgoing veterinarian also has to stretch a bit to match a guarded withdrawn client. This can be done by simply matching body position and perhaps voice volume, slowing down a bit to "join" the client in a manner that is consistent and respectful of his or her communication style.

In Fig. 10, we see the client beginning to speak about her concerns, and the veterinarian is mismatched with her in several ways (ie, the arms crossed, facial expression of coolness, leaning of the body), all of which is nonverbally communicating a sense of detachment. Yet, as the client's story of a tumor on her animal's face begins to unfold, the veterinarian begins to mirror back that concern in her own face, and the client becomes even more expressive of feelings. In Fig. 11, as the client continues her story, she involuntarily begins to hold her hands in the same way as the veterinarian, indicating a sense of connection with the veterinarian and a desire that it continue.

Another important aspect of matching and leading is that it is occurring all the time. If the veterinarian is not aware of the structure of rapport, clients or staff may lead the veterinarian (unintentionally) into a less useful physical, and thus emotional, state of mind and feelings. Most clinicians experience this frequently: a depressed client or one in a chronic state of anxiety may drain a veterinarian emotionally, who, in turn, leaves the encounter wondering what has happened to his or her initial energetic and optimistic state of mind. Many clinicians may respond by avoiding expression of empathy with a client because of this. Remembering that there are two parts to interactional synchrony, and thus to empathy, however, allows the veterinarian to first join the client in his or her anxiety or sadness or withdrawal by matching voice volume or body position and facial expression. The veterinarian can then begin slowly to lead himself or herself (and probably the client as well) out of that physical state, which may influence the client's emotional expression. For example, if a client is sad or withdrawn with head down and a low voice, the veterinarian can assume a similar stance and voice volume. As the interaction progresses, the veterinarian can begin to raise his or her head slowly and gradually raise the

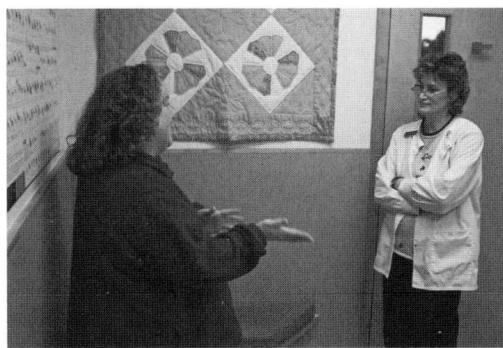

Fig. 10. Developing nonverbal rapport: the veterinarian is mismatched with the client. (Courtesy of Bayer Animal Health Communication Project, New Haven, CT.)

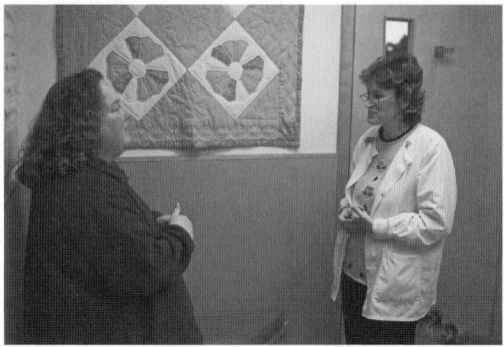

Fig. 11. Developing nonverbal rapport: the veterinarian and client are in interactional synchrony. (Courtesy of Bayer Animal Health Communication Project, New Haven, CT.)

volume of his or her voice. The client is likely to respond in kind and become more engaged in the interaction. The veterinarian then feels a return to a more resourceful state of mind and emotion.

SUMMARY

It is often assumed that skill in nonverbal communication is just "intuition" and that some clinicians have the gift of it and some do not. Nothing could be further from the truth. Treating this more subtle form of interaction with the thoughtfulness and observation with which we approach any other clinical problem can produce a set of skills that can be applied in every encounter. Skill development begins first with enhancing one's observations of nonverbal behavior and then diagnosing whether or not the client is feeling safe. Using one or more of the nonverbal skills when clients are feeling not-safe creates more satisfaction for the client and veterinarian and motivates clients to become full partners in their animal's care.

EXERCISES

Beginning to notice nonverbal behavior consciously takes some practice at first. Develop your sensory acuity in the nonverbal channel by starting small: perhaps for the first several clients on a particular office day, notice voice tonality, rate, and volume. Then, on another day, choose changes in facial color to observe or the way you and the client are positioned in the room with the animal. I used to practice getting into rapport with total strangers on the elevator to my office on the seventh floor of the hospital where I worked, knowing that if I could do it that quickly, I would feel confident about using it in a busy clinical day. Working outside clinical settings is also a good way to practice: when dining out in a restaurant, for example, glance across the room and notice which diners are in rapport and which are not. Watching unscripted television programs for safe and not-safe behaviors, such as talk shows or debates, is also another way to heighten nonverbal awareness.

As you become more comfortable in switching your attention to nonverbal behavior, begin diagnosing those client interactions that are particularly troublesome to you. Begin to notice such things as the following. Does this client seem to be in a safe or a not-safe state? How is the space shaped between us? Are our voices matched in rate or volume? Am I or the client giving a mixed message?

As your nonverbal acuity increases, you naturally find yourself wanting to change your own behavior to create more safety as you interact with your clients. You can be unobtrusive in making some small shifts during the encounter and noticing if your client's behavior changes from a more defensive posture or language to one of greater openness and relaxation.

References

[1] Appendix T. C-6. Basic clinical communication skills. In: Guidelines for bond-centered practice. Fort Collins (CO): Argus Institute, Colorado State University; 2001. p. 1–2.

[2] Lagoni L. Connecting with clients: practical communication techniques for 15 common situations. In: Building the client bond series. Lakewood (CO): American Animal Hospital Association Press; 1998.

[3] Ambady N, Rosenthal R. Thin slices of expressive behavior as predictors of interpersonal consequences: a meta-analysis. Psychol Bull 1992;111(2):256–74.

[4] Beckman H, Markakis K, Suchman T, et al. The doctor-patient relationship and malpractice. Arch Intern Med 1994;154:1365–70.

[5] DiMatteo R, Taranta A, Friedman H, et al. Predicting patient satisfaction from physicians' nonverbal communication skills. Med Care 1980;18(4):376–87.

[6] Argyle M. Spatial behavior. In: Bodily communication. 2nd edition. Madison (CT): International Universities Press; 1988. p. 168–87.

[7] Hall E. Space speaks. In: The silent language. Garden City (NY): Anchor Press; 1973. p. 162–85.

[8] Cassell E. Paralanguage: the music of language. In: Talking with patients, vol. 1: the theory of doctor-patient communication. Cambridge (MA): MIT Press; 1985. p. 10–44.

[9] Carson C. Nonverbal communication. In: Cole S, Bird J, editors. The medical interview: the three-function approach. Philadelphia: Mosby; 2000. p. 225–38.

[10] Lagoni L, Butler C, Hetts S. Nonverbal communication. In: The human-animal bond and grief. Philadelphia: WB Saunders; 1994. p. 118–42.

[11] Hall E. The dance of life. In: The dance of life. Garden City (MA): Anchor Press; 1984. p. 162–4.

Vet Clin Small Anim 37 (2007) 65–77

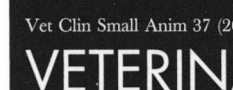

VETERINARY CLINICS
SMALL ANIMAL PRACTICE

Difficult Interactions with Veterinary Clients: Working in the Challenge Zone

James K. Morrisey, DVM[a],*, Bonita Voiland, MS, MBA[b]

[a]Section of Wildlife and Exotic Medicine, Department of Clinical Sciences, College of Veterinary Medicine, Cornell University, PO Box 25, Ithaca, NY 14853-6401, USA
[b]Cornell University Hospital for Animals, Ithaca, NY 14853-6401, USA

As veterinarians, effective interactions with clients and coworkers are fundamental to our professional satisfaction and success. It has been estimated that an average clinician performs more than 100,000 client interactions during his or her career [1]. Undoubtedly, some of these interactions are considered difficult, particularly those involving emotionally laden issues, such as money or euthanasia. This type of interaction may also involve clients labeled as difficult because they are considered overly emotional or the origin of their behavior is not understood.

Regardless of the cause of the difficult interaction, it is important to realize that the problem is in the perception of the interaction and is not necessarily related to any dysfunction of the parties involved. In essence, interactions present as difficult when there is a gap between what is expected to occur and what actually occurs. If we take a step back and look at it as an interaction that requires special attention, the basic rules of good communication covered in previous articles in this issue can help us to address these difficult interactions more effectively. This article first reviews the basis of a difficult interaction and provides specific communication skills to help the veterinarian more successfully manage situations that he or she may find difficult. Then, the authors offer exercises to assist veterinarians in practicing these skills. The information in this article relies closely on the work provided through the Bayer Animal Health Communications Project [2].

Difficult client interactions are inevitable in veterinary practice. This holds true not only for clinicians but for veterinarians involved in administration, research, and the myriad other niches in which veterinarians play important roles. No matter what area of veterinary medicine is practiced, there are interactions with a variety of people, whether they are clients, coworkers, colleagues, or staff, and some of these people may be perceived as "difficult" by you or other coworkers. Although it is common to place blame on other parties involved, it is important to realize that it is the interaction occurring between the

---

*Corresponding author. *E-mail address*: jkm27@cornell.edu (J.K. Morrisey).

parties that is difficult. In the context of clinical care, where there is a tendency to label the client as difficult, it is especially important to recognize this distinction between the interaction and the parties involved. The perspective that classifies the source of difficulty to rest only with the client tends to oversimplify the veterinarian-client relationship, however. Further, this narrow view fails to recognize the diverse variety of factors that have the potential to influence the quality of an interaction, including those surrounding the veterinarian and the practice setting. As the saying goes, "there are two sides to every story"; more aptly, a difficult interaction requires at least two people or parties to occur.

These interactions may start out as difficult but do not have to remain that way. It is important to realize that the interaction is flexible; it is therefore subject to change and can become a more positive interaction. If we think of the difficulty as a function of the individual interaction rather than as a property inherent in one or both parties involved, all that is required is a change in perspective of one or both parties to make the relationship more positive with a more successful outcome. This requires approaching the interaction with an open mind and being willing to demonstrate compassion and to search for understanding.

Furthermore, veterinarians' perceptions about whether an interaction is viewed as difficult are widely variable. Each veterinarian's experiences and expertise contribute significantly to how difficult interactions are managed. As both authors can attest, however, clients who have initially been viewed as difficult have often become the most devoted and enjoyable clients once the cause of the difficulty is understood and acknowledged. Experience and insight can emerge from working through these interactions rather than avoiding them or working around them. It is just like the first time you attempted a procedure, such as a bone marrow aspirate. Initially, it took a great deal of thought and concentration to perform the procedure correctly and efficiently. Each time you performed the procedure, however, you began to gain a greater sense of mastery. As with all skills, communication competence comes with information, effective practice, timely feedback, and more effective practice. Even if you already believe you are an effective communicator, mastering a greater range of skills can help you to understand your role better in situations that do not go as expected. For veterinarians who have worked to develop effective client communication skills, pursuing additional training along with self-reflection can provide insight about interactions perceived as challenging, as well as give an opportunity for planning and practicing techniques to improve those interactions. Focusing and practicing on ways of more effectively interacting and responding to difficult situations can lead to more satisfying outcomes. For example, you may find that you have an unproductive pattern of responding to certain situations, such as when working with angry clients. Identifying and replacing old patterns with new more effective habits can lead to more satisfying encounters for you and your clients.

Let us begin by looking at the three factors that contribute to difficult interactions: the client, the veterinarian, and the patient's problem. Each of these factors has its own characteristics, and they can intersect in a variety of ways to make an interaction difficult. The most common difficulties arise from the following three situations:

- Success is frustrated
- Expectations are misaligned
- Flexibility is insufficient

An example of success being frustrated is when the desired outcome (from the veterinarian's or client's perspective) is not being achieved. The illness may be one that is not treatable, or the owner may not be able to afford the best treatment. Whatever the reason, the ability to achieve a successful outcome is hindered. The second area of difficulty arises when the expectations of the client and the veterinarian are not congruent. For example, the veterinarian and client may have different ideas about what is wrong, what needs to be done, and who is ultimately responsible for resolving the problem. The third area is when the flexibility of one or both parties is insufficient. This may stem from a lack of empathy for or understanding of the view point of the other party and the information that person is bringing to the interaction. As mentioned earlier, it is important to approach these interactions with open-mindedness, flexibility, and compassion. In any interaction, but especially in difficult interactions, it is essential to remember the four basic communication skills: open-ended questions, reflective listening, empathy, and nonverbal communication. Paying attention to these core problem areas and using these skills can serve to prevent situations from becoming difficult or can turn a difficult situation into a positive interaction. Let's look more closely at the specific skills involved when a veterinarian finds himself or herself in an interaction labeled as difficult.

THE CHALLENGE ZONE: ADOBE

It is not difficult to imagine the following scenario. A client requests that you declaw her indoor/outdoor 1-year-old cat because it is ruining the furniture. You are opposed to the procedure, fearing that the cat is likely to lose its ability to defend itself while outside. After a couple of questions, you also discover that the client has not tried behavior modification techniques. As you begin to explain some alternatives, the client seemingly explodes at you, demanding that you perform the procedure. You are offended at the tone and volume used by the client, and you find yourself interrupting the client, speaking more loudly than usual, and repeating yourself in an effort to make the client hear your alternatives and reasoning for each. The situation continues to deteriorate, and you feel as if the client is fighting you. How can you get across your points to the client without driving her away?

Most client interactions fall into what is called the "comfort zone." There are some situations that call for a more focused effort to create a good working relationship with a client, however. These types of situations are often referred to as "challenge zones" (Fig. 1). In human medicine, it is estimated that approximately 30% of the physician-patient relationships fall into the challenge zone

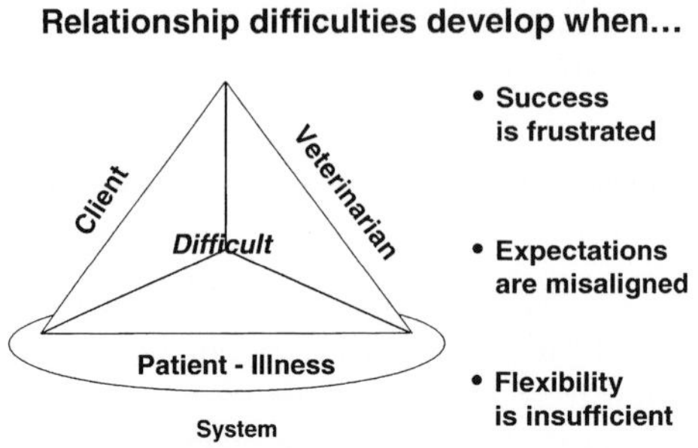

Relationship difficulties develop when...

Client / Veterinarian

Difficult

Patient - Illness

System

- **Success is frustrated**

- **Expectations are misaligned**

- **Flexibility is insufficient**

Fig. 1. Relationship difficulty can come from three sources: the client, the veterinarian, and the patient's problem. The three main areas that can cause difficult interaction are also specified.

category [3]. Beyond the challenge zone is yet another level of complexity—the get-help zone—in which the system in which you are operating needs to be extended even further. Accessing the get-help zone is addressed later in this article.

Studies have shown that successful physicians and other medical professionals often develop defensive behaviors in response to criticism, difficult patient relationships, or patient resistance [4]. The theory is that most health care professionals have little formal training in dealing with this type of situation. Because they have rarely experienced failure, they do not have the skills needed to examine the situation from a neutral perspective and, subsequently, to change their own behavior [5].

Losing your temper or avoiding the situation altogether can have costly results: poor communication and unprofessional behavior increases your chance of ending up in litigation if the case has a poor outcome. [3] More importantly, it can cause clients to seek other veterinarians and can decrease personal satisfaction with your job.

To deal with the situations, the Bayer Animal Health Communication Project uses the mnemonic tool, ADOBE, to assist you in remembering and implementing five categories of actions that can help you to turn difficult situations into more productive relationships (see Fig. 1) [3]. ADOBE stands for the following:

- Acknowledge problems
- Discover meaning
- Opportunities for compassion
- Boundaries
- Extend the system

Acknowledge
The first group of skills involves acknowledging that one or both of you are feeling that the communications between the two of you are not meeting

expectations. This skill group has four components: awareness that a problem exists, assessment about where the problem lies, acceptance of the challenge to fix the problem, and action to build a partnership with the client. Let's review each component in more depth.

The first component of acknowledgment involves awareness that a relationship difficulty exists. For the most part, you are aware when something is wrong because your heightened feelings and internal reactions may be noticeable to you. There are other cues to be aware of that signal the fact that the relationship is in trouble, however. For instance, you may be aware that you are experiencing just an overall feeling of undefined stress, or you may find yourself wishing to end a visit immediately without a clear idea of why. Another common warning sign that the relationship is off-kilter is when you find that you and the client are talking over one another; saying the same things over and over, often louder and louder; and characterizing each other (mentally or out loud) as "one of those kind of people." This is what pediatricians Korsch and Harding [6], authors of *The Intelligent Patient's Guide to the Doctor-Patient Relationship: Learning How to Talk So Your Doctor Will Listen*, call the IRS: interruptions, repetitions, or stereotypic responses.

If you find yourself trying to power through the interaction with the client, take time to step back or pause. If necessary, excuse yourself from the room for a moment to think carefully about why this situation is becoming difficult for you. If it feels as though time is dragging and you are getting bored or tired, this may be a clue that the client is depressed. If you are feeling overwhelmed or irritated, chances are that the client may be feeling the same way. These clues remind you to ask the client how the visit is going for him or her. Commenting on the process of the visit like this can get right to the heart of the matter.

The second component of acknowledging the difficulty is making an assessment about where the problem lies. The model in Fig. 2 addresses the interconnectivity of the dynamics of the situation. First, consider what dimensions are involved: you, the client, or the patient; the illness; the overall system in which the situation is occurring; or a combination of these dimensions. Second, consider what the actual problem is: is a successful outcome not being achieved? In other words, are the expectations of the client (for himself or herself or the animal) or your expectations not being met? How would each of you define success? For the client whose cat requires complex care and attention, success for her may involve not having to worry about injections or a special diet. For you, it may be controlling the signs of the disease.

Are expectations misaligned? Is the difference between your definition of success and that of your client causing problems? Do you share the same understanding of what caused the illness and what should be done about it? You may want to recommend a low-calorie diet for an obese dog that experiences substantial arthritic pain, but your client may think it is cruel to withhold snacks and table scraps.

Is there a lack of flexibility among the various dimensions? Are either or both of you being too inflexible? Can the system be changed to accommodate

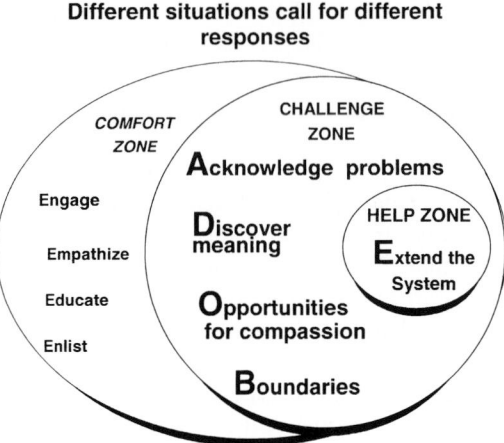

Different situations call for different responses

COMFORT ZONE

CHALLENGE ZONE

HELP ZONE

Engage

Empathize

Educate

Enlist

Acknowledge problems

Discover meaning

Extend the System

Opportunities for compassion

Boundaries

Fig. 2. Veterinarians are comfortable with most aspects of veterinarian-client interactions; however, some interactions fall into the challenge zone as illustrated here. The mnemonic ADOBE can help you to move interactions from the challenge zone back into the comfort zone as discussed in the text.

the problem? Can the client who demands to see his hospitalized bird be provided with some reasonable but limited access? If one or both of you refuse to budge, what are the consequences to the patient?

The third component is accepting the challenge by making a conscious decision to take on the relationship difficulty as thoughtfully as you address the physical aspects of clinical care. If you accept the challenge, you are deciding to take on the care of this patient and that client. You are committing to working on the relationship as well as on the clinical issues. If you do not accept the challenge of working to improve the relationship, what options and obligations do you have for ensuring the patient's care? This situation is more likely in an emergency situation, but it can also happen with clients who have only experienced well-visits before this time.

Assuming that you have assessed the difficulty and accepted the challenge, the fourth component involves acting to build a productive partnership with your client. There are two sides of this action. The first side is to point out your own difficulty with the interaction, and the second is to offer your help. Move the burden of being difficult onto yourself by saying something to the client, for example, "I am having trouble understanding how you'd like me to help," or "I am having trouble knowing how to help because you think I am not responding to your request for declawing your cat. I think it is important for you to fully understand the procedure before you give your permission to have it done." Statements like these are much more helpful than something like "I have a lot of trouble working with people who ask me to declaw their cats."

Another way to acknowledge the problem is by noticing the client's distress: "I can see this visit is not going the way you hoped," or "It looks like you are really upset with me over this." Then follow up with an olive branch, for example, "I would like to work with you, even though we see things differently. Can we plan the next steps together?" Often, shifting your awareness and taking the initial step to bear part of the burden of the difficulty allows the client to do the same, thereby opening both minds to be more willing to accept the changes for a more positive interaction.

Discover Meaning

The second component of the ADOBE model has to do with discovering meaning for the purpose of finding common ground for you and the client. Discovering meaning for the client may require finding out how he or she perceives and whether he or she understands the symptoms or illness of the pet accurately. Before coming to a visit for a problem with their pet, clients have often already done some thinking, Internet researching, worrying, or talking with others about what might be wrong with their animal and what should be done about it. Instead of asking clients what they think is wrong (to which most respond, "I don't know; that's why I came to see you"), ask what they have already learned about the problem or what it is they are most concerned about. It is also helpful to ask what the client expects from you. If you know what the client is thinking, even if it is something you cannot provide or do not want to hear, you have a better chance of explaining your point of view in acceptable terms to the client. For example, a client may demand an MRI scan for her dog, although the clinical indications make MRI a poor diagnostic choice. The veterinarian may believe that he or she is serving the client well by saving her the expense of the MRI scan. The client, conversely, may become angry with the doctor because of the failure to perform an MRI scan, which she honestly believes is going to provide a definitive diagnosis. In this situation, it would help to discover the reason why the client thought an MRI scan was indicated and explain to her why it was not the best medical option.

The visit itself can have meaning, as well. There is an example of a client who treated the staff rudely and was angry even before the technician greeted him. He had brought in his dog for an oncology workup. Nothing the staff could do for this client seemed to make a difference until the veterinarian was able to confront the client gently. He learned that the client's wife had died of cancer just 2 years earlier and that having to bring their dog to the hospital for an anticipated similar diagnosis was almost more than he could bear.

It is also important that you understand the meaning that some illnesses or symptoms have for you. For those of us who have experienced the death of our own companion animal, the first time we see similar symptoms in a client's animal may stir up unexpected emotions. We may respond by backing away from the case or requesting aggressive workups for what seems like a simple problem to the client. How many of us were able to perform our first euthanasia without relating the experience to the euthanasia of one of our own pets when our thoughts and focus should have been on the current client and the patient?

Opportunities to Show Compassion

Understanding what someone else is feeling is essential to creating a good working relationship with a client. Compassion can start with simply being curious about the client's experience with the animal's illness or previous care. Recognizing the emotions behind nonverbal communication and inconsistencies between verbal and nonverbal communication (eg, although verbalizing agreement, a client may be shaking his or her head from side to side indicating "no" or resistance) can further provide insight into the client's feelings. Fear, anger, or sadness can drive clients to repeat themselves until they think they have been heard. All these are clues that the client is anxious.

There are six common ways to express empathy for your client:

- Begin with a review or summary of the events as you understand them. For example, "You called ahead to be sure we were on time because you have to be at work in an hour, and you were left in our reception area for more than 25 minutes past your appointment time without anyone explaining why there was a wait."
- Identify the thoughts and feelings of the client. Continuing with the example, "Because you had called ahead and because we did not let you know that an emergency case came in just before you arrived, you were frustrated with the wait and angry at our inefficiency."
- Verify with the client: "Is that correct?"
- Legitimize thoughts and feelings: "If I were in your shoes, I would feel the same way. I hate waiting, especially when I do not know why I have been left to wait."
- Respect efforts to cope: "Thank you for letting me know that this happened. We are always looking for opportunities to improve our services to clients."

Offer support and partnership: "I would like our team to remember how frustrating it feels when this sort of thing happens. May I use your name and this example in our orientation program? Because you have been such a good client, I think this example might be more effective."

Boundaries

There are four types of boundaries that may need to be adjusted to correct a faltering relationship. These are boundaries related to the following:

- Time: the client's time and the veterinarian's time
- Roles: the client's expectations of the veterinarian's role, the veterinarian's expectation of his or her own role, and the veterinarian's expectation of the client's role
- Content: the words and topics veterinarians talk about with clients
- Physical: space and distance boundaries

First, let us consider the element of time. Difficult relationships take more time because they take more energy. If you can, have clients with whom you have difficult relationships scheduled at a time of the day when you are likely to be relaxed, fresh, and alert. Recognize that most difficult relationships improve slowly and over several appointments, so do not set yourself up for failure by expecting the relationship to turn around after one session. Keep at it.

It's also helpful to remember that no one likes to be kept waiting. Being respectful of a client's time and clients' perception that you may be wasting their time is key. If a delay in services is expected, address the issue promptly and directly. Rather than saying, "We'll be with you in a little while," advise the client that "we are running approximately 45 minutes behind schedule. Would you prefer to wait or reschedule?" If the wait in reception is going to be more than a few minutes, it is also a useful tactic to give clients a clipboard, pencil, and sheet of paper with prompts to guide them to write down the questions they wish to ask the veterinarian and the answers to brief history questions they are likely to be asked.

The next issue to consider involves clarifying and adjusting boundaries related to roles. Although aspects of this have been mentioned previously, it is important to ask what the client expects of the veterinarian and what the client is hoping the veterinarian can do for the animal and client during that visit. If the client has been to a number of veterinarians, ask what works best for the client. If the client's expectations are out of line with your own expectations, address the misaligned expectations directly. Explain what your role is, what you can do, and what can and cannot be accomplished during the visit. This is an important topic and can be at the root of many perceived difficulties with clients. (That is good, because this is often the easiest problem to fix with the simple rules of communication that were mentioned previously.) It is also important to tell clients what you need from them. Repeat that you are interested in caring for the client's animal and that for you to be effective, you are going to need the client's help. Then, spell out what you think you need the client to do, including providing accurate information about the pet, asking for clear explanations, making informed decisions about the care and recommendations, and reporting any changes. Some practices may choose to make these expectations explicit by posting "patient/client rights and responsibilities" in the reception area.

The third boundary to consider is content, meaning what we talk about and the words we use. Initially, you try to open boundaries, learn as much as possible about the client's situation, and reflect on the client's words as much as possible so as to demonstrate empathic understanding. It is important to raise topics that you believe are critical to the care of the patient. In a previous example, had we known that the client had experienced a loss because of cancer in his family, the veterinarian could have said, "This diagnosis of cancer in your pet probably reopens sad memories. Are you concerned in any way about your pet's course of treatment, given what you went through last year?" Simple reflective statements like this can go along way toward bridging the relational gap and strengthening the trust between client and veterinarian.

Equally important to opening boundaries around content is reserving the right to close boundaries around content. In our service-oriented profession, we sometimes forget that we have the right to expect courtesy and respect in return. It is completely within your right to tell a client that you cannot help him or her if he or she uses profanity or is shouting. It is alright to excuse yourself from the room by telling the client it may be beneficial if you both take some time apart to consider the situation. It is acceptable, if a client remains abusive, to ask him or her to leave. No one likes to do this, and it can feel awkward. Being comfortable in the examination room is necessary, however, if you are to continue serving the client. Surprisingly, clients are not offended by this and often respond favorably to this advice. We have found that some clients actually respect the veterinarian more for setting these boundaries and work hard to adhere to them once they understand the established limits of acceptable behavior. In fact, many clients may not be aware of their behavior and modify their behavior promptly when their use of foul language or an abusive tone of voice is addressed.

The final boundary to consider is the physical space and distance between you and the client. People differ in their preference of the personal space they require around them in which to feel comfortable. Be aware that if your client is backing up as you speak to him or her, you are too close. Position yourself so that you can maintain eye contact, and, if at all possible, try to keep your eye level at or a bit below that of the client. Recognize that the examination table or your clipboard can be off-putting barriers or important allies to create needed boundaries. Also, recognize that the safest way to use touch to communicate empathy, warmth, and engagement is to touch the animal. Although a hand on the shoulder or the touch of a client's hand may be a powerful positive communicator, monitor the client's reactions for evidence of discomfort.

Extend the System: The Get-Help Zone

The final technique in ADOBE is called "extend the system." When the relationship simply cannot be mended from within, extending the system means reaching outside the relationship to bring in someone else with a particular skill or expertise. When a relationship is sufficiently difficult so to consider referring the client elsewhere or bringing in help, three questions need to be answered:

- What help is needed? This could be in the form of support, advocacy, expertise, skills, or even legal reporting of an abuse case.
- Who can help and what are the sources? Potential resources can be drawn from family members or friends; other veterinarians or health care professionals; community support services; or local, state, or national agencies, such as adult or child protective services, the local animal shelter, the Humane Society, pastoral services, community mental health services, or suicide prevention programs. It is a good idea to compile a list of these types of resources in advance so that they are readily available when needed.

- How is the client involved in the decision to get help? Ask the client what resources he or she has, what resources the client is currently accessing, and what resources he or she would consider using. Clarify how you would or would not continue to have contact with the client, and agree on how you are going to proceed. If you are not going to have future contact with the client, be sure that the client knows you plan to provide adequate follow-up for the patient's medical care. If you must report abuse, inform the client of the legal requirements and your intention to report the case.

How these questions are answered determines the path the interaction follows. If the relationship progresses and the client's and veterinarian's needs are being met, a positive interaction is likely to ensue. If the client is referred elsewhere for care, the veterinarian knows that he or she has tried everything and that the needs of the animal, client, and doctor are best met by ending the relationship. This is not a failure; it is simply an acknowledgment about what is best for the parties involved.

EXERCISES FOR DIFFICULT INTERACTIONS

Now that you have read about the aspects of dealing with difficult interactions, it is time to practice what you have learned. These exercises are purposefully simple and can be modified to help you gain skill mastery. Applying the skills you have learned and receiving direct constructive feedback about your skills so that you can improve over time is one of the most effective methods of learning. It is much easier to practice new skills in a safe environment with friends or colleagues before trying to use them in a situation in which your own emotions and those of the client are at play. At this point, you may already know which interactions are most difficult for you. If you are uncertain about the areas in which your skills could be improved, ask a coworker whom you trust; such people are often aware of situations that create the greatest anxiety for you and the rest of the veterinary team.

To do these exercises, you need at least two people to help you; thus, you may consider doing these as part of a staff meeting at work. It helps not only to bring you all closer as coworkers but to reaffirm the commitment of the practice to help its clients to the best of its abilities. One person plays the role of the veterinarian, one of the client, and one or more as the observer(s). It is best to have the observer as a separate individual so that the client can really concentrate on his or her role to make sure that the responses are in-line with the character of the client or situation being portrayed. If you find that role playing is difficult or distracting for your group, exercise 2 may help you to formulate answers and "sound bites" for various difficult interactions without having to portray the whole interaction.

Exercise 1
Discuss with your "client" the role you would like the person to play. Be as specific as possible; if you are coworkers, you can draw on a real client scenario, as appropriate. Some examples of possible difficult interactions are given

in Box 1 if you want to practice on a variety of subjects. Discuss with the observer what specific aspects of the communication you would like to work on so that he or she knows what to look for. Give yourself a time limit, such as 3 to 5 minutes, so that the role play provides enough dialogue to examine gaps in communication skills yet does not become repetitive, where the parties lose interest. Now, tell yourself what specific difficulties you may experience with this scenario, and rehearse (in your head or aloud) some of the words you plan to use to turn what would be a difficult interaction into a positive interaction. Although it may seem awkwardly funny at first, try to behave as if this is a real client you are interacting with, because practicing these steps is the best way to make them become part of your communication skill set.

Once you have completed the 3- to 5-minute interaction, make sure that you have at least as long, if not longer, for debriefing. Debriefing is the time for you to get and give feedback on how the exercise worked. All three individuals can take turns describing what specific portions of the dialogue went well or what could have been improved on. The observer can start, because he or she is aware of the specific goals of the exercise for the "vet" in the situation. Once you have finished debriefing, switch roles with a similar client or a new client type. Repeat so that each person has an opportunity to be the veterinarian, the client, and the observer.

Box 1: Some examples of interactions often perceived as difficult

Client unhappy because pet is not improved

Client is angry (reason unknown)

Client is very upset and crying (may be related to pet's illness or more personal in nature)

Client is non-communicative or answers with monosyllabic responses

Client is continually interrupting you to ask questions as you speak

Client has brought spouse or partner and they are giving conflicting information or arguing with one another over the pet

Client disagrees with your diagnosis based on information recovered from the Internet or a friend

Client is unable to decide on course of treatment

Client is sad or frustrated because he/she can't afford the best treatment

Client speaks very loudly (not out of anger, but normal for this client)

Client feels the veterinarian isn't seeing his/her point of view or isn't listening to him/her

Client wants a test or treatment that the veterinarian feels is unnecessary or potentially harmful

Client is upset with negative consequence of a test or diagnostic procedure despite warnings that this could occur

Client makes inappropriate personal statements

Exercise 2

Using an example from Box 1 or developing one of your own, you are now going to practice with at least one other person using specific wording when communicating in a particular difficult client scenario. Provide a brief written description of the scenario, and include the actual words that might be spoken by the client. The first person with the paper should write as if he or she were the veterinarian and write the exact words the veterinarian would use to acknowledge the problem and discover the meaning of the difficult interaction. The paper is then passed to the next person, who responds beneath it using the words he or she would expect the client to use to respond to what the veterinarian has written in the space above. Now, hand the paper to the next person (it may be the first person if only two of you are doing this exercise), and then respond as the veterinarian. Continue this process for several passes until everyone has had at least one chance to write a communication. Now, someone should read aloud the words that have been written based on the client scenario that was agreed on. Read through the entire communication, and then stop and debrief as done in the previous exercise. Everyone should have a chance to say what they think was done well and what they think could be done better. Feel free to let a conversation about this type of interaction flow from this discussion.

References

[1] Bayer Animal Health Faculty Development Program. New Haven (CT); June 9–13, 2003.

[2] Bayer Animal Health Faculty Development Program. The eye of the beholder: difficult interactions between clients and veterinarians. Las Vegas (NV); February 19–20, 2005.

[3] Pichert JW, Miller CS, Hollo AH, et al. What health professionals can do to identify and resolve patient dissatisfaction. Joint Commission on Quality Improvement 1998;24: 303–12.

[4] White MK, Keller VF. Difficult clinician-patient relationships. Journal of Clinical Outcomes Management 2001;8:21–5.

[5] Argyris C. Teaching smart people how to learn. Harv Bus Rev 1991;69(3):99–109.

[6] Korsch BM, Harding C. The intelligent patient's guide to the doctor-patient relationship: learning how to talk so your doctor will listen. New York: Oxford University Press; 1997.

Vet Clin Small Anim 37 (2007) 79–93

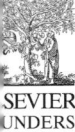

VETERINARY CLINICS
SMALL ANIMAL PRACTICE

Talking with Veterinary Clients About Money

Donald J. Klingborg, DVM[a],*, Jon Klingborg, DVM[b]

[a]Center for Continuing Professional Education, School of Veterinary Medicine, University of California at Davis, One Shields Avenue, Davis, CA 95616, USA
[b]Valley Veterinary Clinic, Merced, CA 95340, USA

WHY DISCUSS MONEY?

Clients seek our services to help preserve the relationship with their animal; improving the life of the animal improves the life of the client. Helping animals, promoting client satisfaction, and generating the financial resources required for a rewarding career are compatible and attainable goals. As veterinarians, we understand that a fair fee for our medical services enables us to deliver quality patient care by providing adequate support for staff and allowing for investment in new medical technology, modernization of facilities, and maintenance of professional competency.

Clients are legitimately interested in the options available for medical care, and understanding these alternatives and associated fees is a vital component of good decision making. In the veterinary setting, the client is purchasing our time, knowledge, and expertise. Clients need to trust the doctor and medical team and want a clear understanding of why they need to do something, what they are getting for their money, when they need to take action, and how the various options minimize whatever risks they perceive.

PROVIDING VALUE TO WHOM?

Veterinary care is a bargain and comprises only a small portion of the total costs associated with animal ownership [1]. Stating this fact does not effectively justify our fees to the client, however. A multiyear study of some 30,000 veterinary clients found that 92% were satisfied with the service they received and 88% indicated that their veterinarian met or exceeded their expectations (Greg Pitto, personal communication, 2004). Yet, only 69% indicated they received sufficient value for the price they paid. A client's recognition of value is based on our ability to communicate with him or her in a manner that makes our efforts appreciated and significant [2].

Let there be no confusion—the key to delivering quality patient care has less to do with our medical skills and more to do with our client skills. Although

*Corresponding author. E-mail address: djklingborg@vetmed.ucdavis.edu (D.J. Klingborg).

0195-5616/07/$ – see front matter
doi:10.1016/j.cvsm.2006.09.007

our interests and talents may be focused on animals, what we are allowed to do and how we generate the revenue needed to invest in our practice are controlled by our clients. Successfully discussing financial matters with clients is an essential step in our career-long journey to deliver optimal patient care.

WHY DO MONEY DISCUSSIONS FEEL SO UNCOMFORTABLE?

In our society, the topic of money has been accurately described as "the last taboo" [3]. Even those physicians who say they feel confident when discussing extremely personal issues with patients (including lifestyle choices involving risky drug, alcohol, and sexual behaviors) report discomfort when discussing the costs of health care [4].

There are several reasons for our collective discomfort. First, our sociocultural heritage includes a fundamental aversion to discussions involving money, sex, and death [5]. As a consequence, clients, doctors, and medical staff all have limited life experience in talking about money. Furthermore, our society attaches strong and highly personal symbolic meaning to money. This personal definition of "meaning" influences how we talk about and spend money and, just as importantly, how we do not [2].

Second, doctors see themselves as healers and believe that discussing money clashes with the goal of helping patients [3]. In today's health care environment, doctors scramble to attend to all their patients and do not want to dilute the limited time available with discussions about nonclinical issues [1]. Many doctors believe that frank discussions about money may raise potential questions about conflict of interest and the doctors' motives for recommending certain diagnostic and therapeutic plans [3]. These concerns are intensified in veterinary medicine, where we proudly embrace the value, "We're veterinarians because we love animals" [6]. We know that clients expect us to demonstrate affection for their animal, and we fear that financial discussions may somehow diminish the perception of our love for and dedication to animals.

Finally, doctors may lack the business skills necessary to engage confidently in informed discussion about fees [4]. Many are unaware of the actual fees associated with a given service or how their overall fee schedule was developed. Some professionals recognize short-term gains to assigning staff the responsibility of presenting estimates, negotiating alternatives, and finalizing payment plans, without consideration of the potential long-term consequences of abdicating this responsibility.

CLIENTS WALK WITHOUT MONEY TALK

In a physician's study of patient preferences, 63% reported a desire to talk with their doctor about fees but only 15% did so [4]. The more direct and forthright style of communication in veterinary medicine is likely to increase the percentage of clients who talk with us about money, but there remain many clients who want to talk money yet do not. Some veterinarians advocate a system in which they agree on a tentative plan of action with the client and staff members prepare and present the fee estimate. Anecdotal reports suggest that this system results in higher client acceptance of the veterinarian's recommended preventive, diagnostic, or therapeutic plan (Carol Schubert, RVT, CVPM, MBA, personal communication, 2004). This approach limits communication and raises concerns about whether the doctor or client is making the decisions about health care. Except in those cases in which the humane care of animals is an issue, the client has the legal authority to make the decision about his or her animal's medical care. Clients differ in their relationships with animals, and the financial limits they place on veterinary care reflect their personal values, beliefs, and economic realities.

The most effective health care providers create functional partnerships with their clients. Clients in challenging situations need to feel supported as much as they need solutions [7]. When the doctor integrates the discussion about clinical alternatives and their associated fees, he or she demonstrates a level of caring for the animal while sending an equally strong message of caring about the client. The integrated discussion also decreases the focus on fees by making money a part of the complete conversation. Creating expectations for clients according to the veterinarian's personal values and failing to charge a fair fee for professional services result in frustrated and unfulfilled practitioners at greater risk for stress and career burnout.

The good news is that the profession is well placed to improve our conversations about the difficult subject of fees. Veterinarians have solid client relationships founded on high levels of trust and a framework for crafting our communication about money based on our experience with the similarly difficult and emotional conversation of euthanasia.

ENGAGING CLIENTS

We intuitively know that few of our clients wake up in the morning and think, "Today I want to go to my veterinarian and spend money." Rather, clients come to us because they receive a benefit when we prevent, diagnose, or treat disease in their animal. Although we, as doctors, tend to think of risks in terms of the likelihood and severity of a disease, clients' perceptions of risk are more subjective. Their reactions can include feelings of outrage and injustice because of the need to face the animal's medical problem and fear associated with the loss of their investment of emotion, time, and money [8]. As clinical practitioners, we have all experienced exaggerated client responses to a perceived crisis, including critical and emotional reactions; rejection of reasonable and justified medical plans; denial accompanied by agitation and disbelief; and even avoidance, withdrawal, and hopelessness [8]. Although the client's perceived risk may not represent the true risk as we know it, the risk is "real" to the client, and it is essential that we acknowledge and address these concerns (W. Hueston, P. DeVito, P. Sandman, S. Annette, National Center for Food Protection and Defense, University of Minnesota, personal communication, 2006).

In low-stress situations, such as a routine physical examination or vaccination, clients primarily make decisions based on their perception of the veterinary professional's expertise and competency. Contrast that with high-stress situations, such as catastrophic and life-threatening illness or injury, where clients evaluate a veterinary professional first on his or her capacity to listen, care, and empathize; then on honesty and openness; and, finally, on expertise and competence. Clients in distress need to know that you care before they care what you know. Highly stressed clients judge the messenger before they judge the message, and their evaluation is based primarily on whether or not they trust you.

Trust grows from a belief that you are on their side. Learn to mirror their emotion, convey your concern and empathy, listen to how they feel, and determine what they need. Accept the uncertainty of the situation, and do not over-reassure. Do not leave a vacuum of information, because clients quickly fill any gaps in their understanding from other (less reliable) sources. Accept that it is normal and acceptable for clients to be afraid, even if your opinion is that their fear is unjustified. Tell them what you know, what you do not know, and how you recommend going about finding the missing answers. Avoid absolute statements, such as "always" or "never," because even one exception proves you wrong. Recognize that people's levels of distress are based on a variety of assessments (Table 1), including whether a particular threat is natural or not. An accidental poisoning of an animal, for instance, does not provoke the same intensity of feelings experienced with an intentional poisoning. Understanding the situation may help you to understand the client's perspective and the reasons for his or her responses or behavior. Clients are not children; treat them with respect and as partners in the journey toward better health for their animal.

Table 1
Responses to various types of risks

Lower feelings of outrage and dread	Higher feelings of outrage and dread
Voluntary	Involuntary
Lung cancer in a smoker	Lung cancer from second-hand smoke
Personally controlled	Controlled by others
Intoxicated or speeding driver in accident	Victim of a drunk driver or speeder
Familiar	Exotic
Influenza, cancer	SARS, bird flu
Natural	Man made
Creutzfeldt-Jakob disease	v-Creutzfeldt-Jakob disease (mad cow)
Reversible	Permanent
Fracture	Amputation
Fairly distributed	Unfairly distributed
Loss of life in tornado	Inability for those in poverty to evacuate Hurricane Katrina
Affects adults	Affects children
Quick and relatively painless death	Slow agonizing death

Complied by the authors using materials developed by the US Center for Disease Control and Prevention and from lecture materials developed by Will Hueston, Paul DeVito, Vincent Covel, and Peter Sandman.
Abbreviation: SARS, systemic acute respiratory distress syndrome.

"BECAUSE I SAID SO"

The terms *compliance* and *adherence* have been hot topics in health care over the past few years and affect the health of patients, the timely use of professional services, and money. In general, the terms refer to clients' acceptance of and success in following their doctor's recommendations and instructions. The data in human and veterinary medicine are clear—people are failing to follow preventive, diagnostic, and therapeutic plans as prescribed by their doctor. A 2003 survey of veterinary clients found 52% of those surveyed to be out of compliance with heartworm preventive, 65% with dental prophylaxis, approximately 65% with senior health screening, and approximately 80% with prescription diets [9]. The reasons relate to a communication disconnection between the doctor's suggestions for best patient care and clients' understanding of how the money and effort requested ultimately benefit them.

Compliance and adherence fail to capture the nature of the doctor-client relationship. They imply that the doctor is the dominant authority, who tells the client what to do. This survey and similar surveys in human medicine demonstrate with clarity that the authority to decide what is and is not done resides with the client. The difference between following or ignoring the doctor's medical advice is associated with a commitment, freely given, by the client. This commitment results from education and negotiation rather than from coercion or direction or by providing limited options.

Motivation is internally driven and built on understanding why something needs to be accomplished, what and when it needs to be done, and how the client can successfully complete the necessary tasks. We have all told clients to "give two tablets twice a day and return in 2 weeks for a recheck," only to have them return for an unrelated issue several weeks later with tablets left over. Successfully negotiating a commitment requires meeting the needs of all parties and depends on the doctor actively listening to clients to determine their interests. Interest-based negotiations create win-win outcomes and acknowledge that there are several satisfactory solutions to every problem. When challenged by a client holding an inflexible position, look for interests that overlap the client's position and your advice. Negotiating is simply determining how value is distributed between the parties and depends on demonstrating how the client receives benefits from the solution.

The "because I said so" argument inherent in compliance and adherence was ineffective when our parents used it on us as children and has no place in doctor-client communications.

ACQUIRING YOUR SERVICES

When faced with the need for catastrophic medical intervention for their animal, clients often are confronted with a financial dilemma. As the technical experts, it is our responsibility to help clients break through their budgetary "glass ceiling" and find ways for them to pay for the necessary veterinary services. Doing so maintains our relationship with their animal and results in treatment rather than euthanasia.

It is common today to hear financial consultants lecture about the evils of extending credit to clients and the benefits of accepting only cash, checks, and credit cards. External credit services have grown rapidly by providing funds that enable clients to pay for the necessary services. These businesses have been successful because they have captured the loan fees and interest that once went to the practice, and they have benefited from the low failure-to-pay rate that exists in veterinary medicine (Lou Gatto, CPA, personal communication, 2003). All practices have had clients who did not pay their bills, but practices that do not allow the occasional delinquent client to frame his or her credit policy are likely to find that most clients do pay.

Financially successful veterinary practices have the resources necessary to support best patient care and benefit from a combination of four business variables: controlling expenses, attracting more client visits, providing more necessary services per client visit, and collecting higher fees for a given service. Most practice management advice focuses on optimizing the last three variables. Success in these areas begins with helping clients to get what they want rather than with the practice trying to get what it wants. Achieving success with clients involves open communication, including understanding the client's desires through active listening, allowing the client to make the best decision for himself or herself by providing information and options, and positioning the practice team to be supportive and nonjudgmental.

THE MESSAGE

Veterinarians cannot fail to communicate. Every aspect of every interaction with a client communicates something. Even silence, such as failing to respond during a conversation or to return a telephone call, leaves a void the client is likely to fill with speculation, assumptions, and misperceptions. Successful veterinarians create positive messages, understand their role as the messenger, and deliver information in a way that affects health care outcomes.

Effective messages describe, in order of importance, the payoff (goal), purpose (why), action (what), timing (when), and process (how). The most effective messages describe the payoff in terms that are directly relevant to the client. Focus the conversation on how the animal is likely to benefit (goal) rather than emphasizing veterinary services, facilities, and equipment (how).

Trust is built through interaction; thus, clients need to work with you before they are ready to purchase your services [6]. Make an effort to become associated with good news. Physicians regularly mail normal test results to patients, missing the opportunity to strengthen the relationship with the patient by delivering and celebrating the results with the patient. Veterinarians tend to be apologetic if a test they suggested does not lead to a definitive diagnosis. Frame messages about negative tests as positive outcomes by saying something like, "This is great news; we've ruled out XYZ disease, have a future benchmark for organ function in your animal, and are narrowing the possible causes of the clinical signs."

Solutions only count if people know that they have a problem. Explain the problem and how it may affect the animal. Develop messages from an understanding that people desire to preserve the known or familiar, and strive first to avoid making a bad choice and only then look toward making the best choice. Compare and contrast the risk the client perceives with the various options for care by prioritizing the problem list and moving the focus to the most medically important [10].

Deliver information by using comparisons between the patient's current status and alternative approaches, for example, "Rover is getting around but can no longer get on the couch or climb the stairs. There isn't much we can do to reverse his arthritis, and the medication available has some risks we'll discuss further. There is a very good chance, however, that medication will alleviate most of the pain he's currently experiencing and improve his ability to do those things he loves." Organize your messages to "stop the pain" before discussing "delivering the gain."

People differ, and the effectiveness of a message differs with them. Men tend to be more visual than women and relate better to images, charts, and models [11]. Women tend to be more averse to risk and pragmatic, are less likely to accept some interventions, and often prefer more information and time to make medical decisions. Women were willing to spend more than men if the chance of their animal's recovery was 75% and less than men if the chance of recovery was 10%. Men and women had lower spending limits for cats as compared with those for dogs [12]. Preferred styles of communication also vary between individuals independent of gender, and a helpful summary of some key differences and approaches is presented in Table 2.

Discussing fees is different from discussing your expenses. Avoid the common trap of trying to evoke sympathy and understanding from your clients by explaining your expenses as a means to justify your fees. Clients are interested in themselves and their reality and not in your financial situation. Most clients overestimate your income and perceive that you have an easier life than they do. Discussing your expenses simply makes you look unprofessional and raises doubts about your motives.

Your requests should be worded to demonstrate that you are interested in answering the often unspoken client question "Why should I?" For example, use such phrases as the following: "To help you save time, please fill out these forms...," "To minimize your expenses, please pick your animal up by 6:00 PM today," and "To help me quickly complete your prescription request, please provide the following information..."

Estimates can be powerful messages for clients and are best organized by grouping expenses into categories rather than detailing each item or service and its associated fee. Providing too much detail overwhelms the client, delivers information he or she cannot interpret, and creates numerous targets that might spur disagreement. Disagreement with even one item on your detailed list may be enough for the client to assume that all the charges are questionable [4].

Table 2
Client preferences for effective communication styles[a]

	Cows	Dogs	Cats	Horses
	Organized, process oriented	Relationships, people oriented	Idea oriented, analytic	Action oriented, free spirited
Want to know	Why and what	Who and how	Why and how	What and who
Personality styles				
Basic needs	Order	Honesty	Rationality	Freedom from control by others
Expectations	Judgment	Emotional involvement	Logic	Sensation
Learn best by presentations that are	Organized, practical, concrete	Enthusiasm, participatory	Data based, analytic interpretation	Hands on, interactive, include models and physical contact
Troubled by	Disorder, instability	Dishonesty, lack of feelings	Sentimentality and lack of logic	Authority, pomposity
Communication Styles				
Opening preferences	Precise facts	Engage relationship before discussing issues	Make connection to larger medical concepts	Results of actions
Statements	Logical order	Focused on the client's relationship with the animal	How the problem uniquely affects the patient	Prefer recommendations with few alternatives
Emphasis	Options with pros and cons	How alternatives have worked in other patients	Results, future expectations for performance	Practicality of recommendations and expected outcomes
Time sensitivity	Slowest assimilation and consideration		Slow and careful approach	Rapid assimilation preferring brief presentation
Helped by	Outlines of proposal	References to recognized authorities	Reviewing key concepts	Visual aids, charts, models

[a]Each person is a unique combination of the four columns, and these styles denote only preferences and do not define who we are.
Data from Maddrone T. Living your colors: practical wisdom for life, love, work and play. New York: Warner Books; 2002; and Carlson Learning Company. DiSC dimensions of behavior. Minneapolis (MN): Carlson Learning Company; 1994; and Youker R. Communication styles instrument: a teambuilding tool. In: Anderson RJ, editor. Personal Medical Information First International Workshop Proceedings. Cambridge (UK): Springer-Verlag; 1996. p. 796. Available at: web.mit.edu/mbarker/www/pmi96/commp796.txt. Accessed January, 2006.

Send a message that says "thank you," and mean it. Clients and their animals are the reason why there is a veterinary profession and why you are in business. They have done you a tremendous service by trusting the care of their animal to you. Clients want to feel validated that they are taking good care of their animal. By seeking your expertise, they have taken a significant step toward that good care. Make sure that you help them to feel good about the choices they make for their animal. Many businesses go beyond thanking them at the point of service and send cards around Thanksgiving or during National Pet Week. What are you doing to say "thank you" to your clients?

THE MESSENGER

Doctors set the pace and the mood in their practice every day. "Staff infection" is contagious and spreads directly from the doctor's attitude. Clients pick up cues from doctors and staff about the necessity and value of products and procedures. Veterinarians need to be able to explain how their services and products provide value to clients and patients. They need to convince themselves and their staff that recommendations are appropriately based on the patient's condition and that fees are fair to clients and the practice. A common understanding and commitment within the entire medical team are essential for consistent and believable messages to be delivered to clients.

There are major financial differences between non-for-profit organizations and private veterinary practices (although many of the latter operate as if they are not-for-profit organizations). Profit is fundamental if you plan on providing the best patient care throughout your career. How to create fair profits within your practice is beyond the scope of this article, but it is essential that veterinarians and their staff accept the direct relation between profit and best patient care. Those unable to make this connection are not able to justify fees to others and may be better suited for careers in a not-for-profit setting.

Clients judge you quickly and by a variety of cues. Within a minute of your entry into the examination room, they have formed perceptions about your personality, sophistication, trustworthiness, sense of humor, social heritage, education level, career competence, and success [12]. Much of their evaluation is based on your appearance and body language, less on how you sound, and still less on the words you use to communicate. Look and act professionally. Put a mirror outside each examination door, and check yourself before you enter. Change dirty smocks and comb your hair before entry. Wash you hands or use a rinse-free antiseptic for your hands in the presence of the client when you enter the examination room. Leave the mental clutter and frustration of your day behind when you walk through the door and greet the client. Clear your mind. Focus completely on your client during your time together, and make it your sole mission to help that client and patient. Building rapport, setting the agenda, exchanging information, responding to emotions, detecting cues, reaching common ground, and agreeing on next steps are milestones in every client interaction.

Provide information to enable the client to make an informed decision rather than trying to coerce behavior that meets your values or needs. The use of coercive or dominant power results in greater distancing between the doctor and client, greater distrust, and the attribution of negative qualities to the dominating party while holding one's self in higher esteem. In contrast, the use of informal power, including information, expertise, and goodwill, builds positive relationships [13].

FEES

Most fee schedules evolve from some historical precedent that may or may not have reflected true expenses or included a fair profit margin. Setting fees ideally involves an accounting for the true costs of doing business, including evaluating current expenses associated with supplies, time, technology, facility space, insurance, breakage or loss, and other expenses, before adding a fair profit. This method is time-consuming and difficult. Most practices take a simpler route, periodically updating their current fee structure with a percentage increase based on cost-of-living data (inflation rates or consumer price indices). The cost of some products changes rapidly, and to maintain profitability, it is critical for fees related to those products to follow suit.

Remember that fees regularly include expenses that are not part of a specific procedure. Human hospitals historically have applied a multiple to the actual costs of the medical procedure. The total fee charged includes expenses associated with the service or procedure, malpractice insurance, billing costs and revenue delays associated with insurance and to cover the costs of indigent care (David Baum, personal communication, 2001).

Uniqueness and reputation allow for higher fees, and competition tends to lower fees. Higher fees may be justified if you provide a unique service in your competitive region because you have special training and expertise, an exclusive piece of medical technology, or a widespread reputation for excellence in a specific procedure. Fees often include a subjective bias, with many doctors discounting their fees for those procedures they especially enjoy and charging well above fair market value for those they prefer to avoid.

The fees associated with office calls, spays or neuters, nails or ears, parasite control, dental prophylaxis, vaccination, and prescription diets are directly competitive within your service area and are frequently telephone-shopped by clients (Lou Gatto, personal communication, 2004). Other services are more difficult to compare and are not as sensitive to competition. When a client calls and asks how much a cat spay costs, make sure that he or she receives the answer that differentiates your higher fee from the competition by explaining the uniqueness and value of your service. Simply to quote the higher fee sends most shoppers elsewhere, because the client did not learn why your service was superior and worth the higher fee.

Get comfortable charging for your expertise. Charging for services is part of the rite of passage to becoming a true professional [3]. Benchmarking fees is a valuable management technique and recommended as part of a fee review.

Table 3 provides some local benchmarking comparisons to help remind you of the comparative value of your time and expertise. Create your benchmarking comparison by completing Table 3 with information from your practice and by gathering local fees from other service providers as suggested in Table 3. Refer to other resources from organizations and in journals to benchmark your fees for service.

Be direct, explicit, and nonapologetic about your fees. Present your recommendation pleasantly and wait for the client's reply: "I'm suggesting the best medical care I know of for your animal's condition. Let me know if expense is an obstacle and we'll explore less costly alternatives." If the client remains undecided, ask what may be delaying a decision and fill the information gap.

Table 3
Benchmarking to convince veterinarians and staff that it is okay to charge for professional services

Occupation	Education/training	Ask them

Veterinarian	Avg 8.5 years of college
	National and state
	  licensing examinations
	Continuing education
		Charge for physical
		  examination and
		  how long it takes
		  ($/examination ×
		  number/hour =
		  hourly rate)

Physical
  therapist
	Master's degree
	National and state
	  licensing examinations
	Continuing education
		Charge for 1 hour
		  of therapy

Plumber	Apprenticeship
	Certification courses
	May have licensing tests
		House call fee
		  and hourly
		  rate to replace a
		  water heater or
		  repair a faucet,
		  not including
		  materials

Electrician	Apprenticeship
	Certification courses
	May have licensing tests
		House call fee and
		  hourly rate to install
		  a new electrical outlet,
		  not including materials

Auto
  mechanic
	6 months to 2 years
	Certification
	  courses by subject
		Hourly shop fee for
		  changing oil and filters,
		  not including materials

Auto body
  craftsman
	6 months to 2 years
	Certification
	  courses by subject
		Hourly shop fee for
		  repairing a fender,
		  not including materials

Dog groomer	On-the-job training
	  2–18 week's of
	  educational programs
	No licensing in
	  most states
		Standard fee to clip a
		  dog and how long it
		  takes (average ~2 hours)

THE DELIVERY

You cannot bore people into trusting you or taking your advice. The messenger needs to deliver the message enthusiastically, professionally, and, hopefully, with conviction. This means you need to invest time and effort in preparing yourself to communicate effectively by using language that the client understands. Accept the role of guide and resource expert, and navigate rather than drive the interaction. Embrace the veterinarian's role to interpret, translate, educate, and facilitate the decision about the medical options available to meet the patient's needs.

The malpractice suit is the ultimate example of a messenger failing to deliver the message. Levinson [14] recorded hundreds of conversations between physicians and patients. Half of the doctors had never been sued; the other half had been sued at least twice. The differences were in how they talked with their patients. Surgeons who were never sued spent approximately 3 minutes longer with each patient (18.3 versus 15 minutes) and were more likely to have made orienting comments, such as "First, I'll examine you, and then we'll talk about what I found and provide time to answer your questions." Those not sued were more likely to engage in active listening; to make comments, such as "Go on, tell me more about that...," and laughed more during the visit. There were no differences in the amount of "quality medical information" shared.

As a follow-up, a psychologist examined the recordings, masked the actual words by removing the high-frequency sounds that make words recognizable, and left the lower frequency sounds that reflect "feelings." By quantifying warmth, hostility, dominance, and anxiousness, the psychologist was able to predict accurately which surgeons were sued.

Clients need to feel respected and supported. In another study, it was found that 40 seconds of empathetic conversation reduced cancer patients' anxiety and increased the perception of the caring nature and helpfulness of the doctor [15]. Pay attention to the feelings you express to clients. Make and review audiotaped recordings of your client interactions. Ask staff for feedback on your delivery, and remember to thank and not shoot the messenger if your staff points out some areas ripe for improvement.

Once you have engaged with the clients, let them know you care about the relationship they have with their animal. Follow the framework for communicating found elsewhere in this article. Recognize that "one size does not fit all" and that clients have different preferences for the way in which information is provided. As the navigator and guide, you have to adapt your presentation to the individual.

When meeting new or anxious clients, it is often helpful to prepare them for the visit by providing a summary of what you plan to do and identify when they can ask their questions. Many veterinarians use a white board in their examination rooms to capture questions as they come up, demonstrating visually that they "heard" the question and plan to address it in due course.

Avoid making assumptions or value judgments about your clients. Clients often communicate their concerns in order of priority, and the most effective doctors continue to ask if there are any other problems or concerns until the client says "No." Ask questions to clarify their meaning, and record and paraphrase a client's comments to demonstrate that you are listening and to confirm that you understood what he or she wants.

Alert clients to what is coming by framing the remarks with comments like "This is good news" or "This concerns me..." Ask them how much detail they want, and provide information in discrete chunks. Use neutral and objective phrases rather than authoritative and value-laden phrases like "you should." Check in with them frequently, for example, "The drug I'm prescribing is expensive but is the best for most patients with this condition. If you decide you can't afford it, let me know, and we'll see if something else will work...Okay?" Wait, watch, listen, and address their response. "No" is not a rejection of you or your plan but rather a gift of information indicating the need for more information.

A "stealth recommendation" is useless to your patients, your clients, and your practice. A recent study demonstrated that most clients did not recognize that their veterinarian had made a recommendation for dental prophylaxis or senior screening [9]. In most cases, a follow-up review of medical records failed to show any recorded recommendation for senior screening. Those few clients who "heard" the recommendation and chose not to accept it did so because they "didn't have time to meet the request," it was "too inconvenient," or they "didn't understand the need." Only a small percentage reported nonacceptance because of the cost, and three of four clients surveyed agreed that vets only recommend products or procedures that are good for their pets. If your clients are missing your recommendations, change your message or delivery. Communicate explicit and specific recommendations, including any options, by alerting them to what is coming (eg, "I recommend...").

Give clients time to assimilate what you have told them and to organize their thinking. Ask them if they need more time before you continue. Teachers recommend allowing a minimum of 6 seconds of silence after asking a question of students (Steven Venette, personal communication, 2006). Six seconds seems like a long time in an examination room, especially when faced with serious health issues. People do, however, process information at different rates of speed, and although the patient's problem may represent familiar territory for the doctors and clinic staff, it likely is new information for the client.

Ask clients what level of detail they prefer for the information you provide. Anticipate that clients may want to discuss a treatment plan's costs and any alternatives. You may not know the fees associated with every portion of the proposed medical plan, but your ability to communicate the range of fees for the average case of parvovirus, fracture, or pyometra, for example, sends a positive message about your knowledge and the value of your services. Provide a maximum of two or three alternatives. Too many options overwhelm and paralyze the decision-making process. Finally, stop offering alternatives once a client has decided on a course of action [7].

There are many different types of clients. The client who responds to your recommendation with an impassive facial expression did not understand you or has not yet developed sufficient trust in you. If a client is indecisive, offer an opportunity to call a spouse, partner, or trusted friend to talk over the options. The Internet is delivering more "informed" clients with medical insight courtesy of surfing good and bad web sites. These clients respond best when you acknowledge and validate their effort at educating themselves. Avoid the "I'm the doctor, and I know more than you" trap. Outline your recommendations, and answer their questions without debating any contrary information they have acquired. If challenged, respond with "In my experience..." or "There are differences in opinions, and I base my recommendations on..."

THE MISSING LINK

A critical step often overlooked in the doctor-client conversation is asking for the sale. It is as simple as saying, "May we initiate the diagnostic or therapeutic process now?" Retailers have long known that customers must perceive that you care enough to sell "it" before they are willing to buy "it." If you do not believe in the value of your services and care enough to ask clients to initiate the diagnostic or therapeutic plan, you cannot expect them to care enough to purchase your services.

To be sure they caught the most important points, ask clients how they plan to share the information with their families and friends when they go home. Help them to organize their thinking and understanding, create clear expectations for how the process is going to unfold, and check in with them about any questions or concerns that have not been answered. Support them with statements about how you plan to partner with them, and ask what you can do to make their experience more comfortable.

SUMMARY

Service is defined by the provider; satisfaction is determined by the client. Every personal interaction, every aspect of your operation, and the entirety of your product or service are considered and weighed by the client against his or her personal value system [2].

Every person associated with the practice is part of the communication team, gathering and recording information on the client's preferences and disseminating information about products and services. The major difference between veterinary clinics is not in the quality of medicine practiced but in how its clients are treated. Embrace the fact that it is not about you and that it is about them. Clients want to preserve the relationship they have with their animal. Effective communication demonstrates your dedication, trustworthiness, professionalism, and concern and is integral to career-long success and satisfaction.

Money is an important part of the conversation and an area in which you can develop expertise equal to your medical skills. The effort is likely to pay significant dividends to your patients, your clients, your practice, and you.

References

[1] Getz M. Veterinary medicine in economic transition. Ames (IA): Iowa State University Press; 1997. p. 3–13.

[2] Sanders B. Fabled service: ordinary acts, extraordinary outcomes. San Francisco (CA): Jossey-Bass; 1997. p. x, 1–13, 44.

[3] Holloway JD. Talking dollars. Money Matters 2003;V1(1):1–2.

[4] Borglum K. Talking with patients asbout costs. Sonoma Medicine 2004;55:1–5. Available at: www.scma.org/magazine/scp/sp04/borglum.html. Accessed January 2006.

[5] Miller M, Mayer K, Makadon HJ. Talking about safer sex with your patients. The Fenway Institute/Fenway Community Health. Available at: www.biresource.org/bothteams/safesexbrochure.html. Accessed January 2006.

[6] Milani MM. The art of veterinary practice: a guide to client communication. Philadelphia: University of Pennsylvania Press; 1995. p. 33, 143–55.

[7] Brem JL. Women make the best salesmen. New York: Currency Doubleday; 2004. p. 131, 174.

[8] Centers for Disease Control and Prevention. The psychology of crisis. The Fenway Institute/Fenway Community Health. Emergency risk communication. Atlanta (GA): Centers for Disease Control and Prevention; 2005. p. 1–6. Available at:www.cdc.gov/communication/cdcynergy_eds.htm.

[9] American Animal Hospital Association and Hill's Pet Nutrition. The path to high-quality care; practical tips for improving compliance. Lakewood (CO): The American Animal Hospital Association; 2003. p. 12–3, 15.

[10] Beckwith H. Selling the invisible, a field guide to modern marketing. New York: Warner Books; 1997. p. 169–214.

[11] Kapral MK, Devon J, Winter AL, et al. Gender differences in stroke care decision making. Med Care 2006;44(1):70–80.

[12] Brown JP, Silverman JD. The current and future market for veterinarians and veterinary medical services in the United States. J Am Vet Med Assoc 1999;215(2):161–83.

[13] Gardner DB. Ten lessons in collaboration. Online J Issues Nurs 2005;10(1):1–17.

[14] Gladwell M. Blink, the power of thinking without thinking. New York: Little, Brown & Company; 2005. p. 41–3.

[15] Fogarty LA, Curbow BA, Wingard JR, et al. Can 40 seconds of compassion reduce patient anxiety? J Clin Oncol 1999;17:371–9.

Vet Clin Small Anim 37 (2007) 95–108

VETERINARY CLINICS
SMALL ANIMAL PRACTICE

End-of-Life Communication in Veterinary Medicine: Delivering Bad News and Euthanasia Decision Making

Jane R. Shaw, DVM, PhD[a,b,*], Laurel Lagoni, MS[c]

[a]Argus Institute, Colorado State University, Fort Collins, CO 80523, USA
[b]James L. Voss Veterinary Teaching Hospital, Colorado State University, 300 West Drake Road, Fort Collins, CO 80523, USA
[c]World by the Tail, Inc., www.PetPeopleHelp.com, 126 West Harvard Street, Suite 5, Fort Collins, CO 80525, USA

W ith increasing recognition of the relationships that people develop with their companion animals [1] comes an awareness of the impact of animal death on pet owners and the veterinary team [2,3]. Rising acknowledgment of pets as family members has been associated with increasing expectations of pet owners for the highest quality medical care for their companion animals as well as compassionate care and respectful communication for themselves [1,4]. Research [2] indicates that 70% of clients are affected emotionally by the death of their pet and that as many as 30% of clients experience severe grief in anticipation of or after the death of their pet. In addition, approximately 50% of clients studied reported feeling guilty about their decision to euthanize their pet. One of the factors contributing to client grief was the perception of the professional support provided by the veterinarian. The manner in which the veterinarian provides care for a client whose pet has died has the potential to alleviate or aggravate grief.

Growing evidence indicates that providing emotional support to pet owners contributes to stress among members of the veterinary practice team [5]. It has been reported that veterinarians are present at the death of their patients five times more often than other health care professionals [6]. Creating a practice culture that promotes self-care and work-life balance is essential to preventing stress, compassion fatigue, and burnout [7,8]. Promoting an atmosphere of collegial support, respect, and empathy serves as the foundation for providing care to clients and their pets.

End-of-life discussions present challenges for veterinarians and clients. From the veterinarian's perspective, a number of factors [9–11] contribute to discomfort,

*Corresponding author. James L. Voss Veterinary Teaching Hospital, Colorado State University, 300 West Drake Road, Fort Collins, CO 80523. *E-mail address*: jane.shaw@colostate.edu (J.R. Shaw).

0195-5616/07/$ – see front matter
doi:10.1016/j.cvsm.2006.09.010

including lack of training, being short of time, practice culture, feeling responsible for the patient's illness, perceptions of failure, unease with death and dying, lack of comfort with uncertainty, impact on the veterinarian-client-patient relationship, worry about the patient's quality of life, and concerns about the client's emotional response and his or her own emotional response to the circumstances. Some of the same reasons [11] account for client anxiety in receiving bad news. These include self-blame, unease with death and dying, anticipatory grief, effect on the human-animal bond, impact on the veterinarian-client-patient relationship, pet's quality of life, and concerns about their emotional response to the situation. Research [9,11,12] in human medicine indicates that end-of-life discussions are often suboptimal because of many of the barriers presented here and lack of specific training in end-of-life communication.

The content, duration, and methods of end-of-life communication training in veterinary curricula are highly diverse and variable. Many practitioners have not received formal training and may feel unprepared to engage in these conversations [13]. Educators have identified a skills gap between the content of the veterinary school curriculum and the actual skills required to be a successful veterinarian [14–16]. Practitioners recognize the importance of interpersonal communication. In alumni surveys, communication skills and dealing with clients were listed as the most important skills for success in veterinary practice [17,18], and interpersonal skills were recognized as the main selection criterion used for selecting new graduates [18]. Surveys [13,19–21] indicate that veterinary students understand the importance of addressing the human-animal bond and the need to provide pet loss support when interacting with clients. Taken together, the results of these surveys demonstrate that veterinary educators, practitioners, and students have a strong interest in incorporating communication skills training into the veterinary curriculum.

Extrapolating from evidence in human medicine, how end-of-life conversations are conducted has the potential to influence clinical outcomes, including the creation of an enduring veterinarian-client relationship and veterinarian and client satisfaction [10–12,22,23]. When end-of-life discussions are conducted skillfully, difficult decisions are validated, clients' concerns are heard, and emotions are supported. If these discussions are executed poorly, however, leading to dissatisfaction with the veterinarian or overall veterinary care, the communication can complicate grief, reduce client compliance and retention, and increase the likelihood of litigation [2,22,24–26]. Conducting compassionate end-of-life discussions has the potential to enhance professional satisfaction and to reduce compassion fatigue and burnout [11].

End-of-life communication in veterinary medicine includes delivering bad news; monitoring and assessing quality of life; euthanasia decision making; discussing the euthanasia protocol and body care options; and providing grief support, education, and resources. The purpose of this article is to present best practices for delivering bad news and euthanasia decision making. There are limited empiric studies in the veterinary literature concerning veterinarian-client-patient communication, and information pertaining specifically to end-of-life conversations is based largely on clinical experience [22]. In human medicine, studies of end-of-life communication are based primarily on expert opinion, case studies, reviews, and predominantly descriptive studies [12,27]. In this article, the SPIKES six-step model (setting, perception, invitation, knowledge, empathize, and summarize), developed by Buckman [11] and currently employed in medical curricula, is utilized to structure end-of-life conversations in veterinary medicine.

UNDERLYING PREMISES

Three underlying principles guide communication skills training in end-of-life conversations:

1. Given the expectations of clients and the impact of end-of-life conversations on pet owners and the veterinary team, compassionate communication is considered to be an ethical obligation, a core clinical skill, and integral to the success of a veterinary team [2,3,28,29].
2. End-of-life communication is related to significant clinical outcomes, including enduring veterinarian-client-patient relationships and veterinarian and client satisfaction [10–12,22,23].
3. Effective techniques for end-of-life communication can be taught and are a series of learned skills. Communication skills can be delineated, defined, and measured, and these skills are best learned through observation, well-intentioned and descriptive feedback, and repeated practice and rehearsal of skills [30].

THE GRIEF PROCESS

Before engaging in end-of-life conversations with clients, it is helpful to gain a basic understanding of the normal grief responses and processes [3,31]. Symptoms of grief can range from stoicism to sobbing or even intense anger. Although deep expressions of grief can be difficult to witness, these emotions are a necessary and natural part of emotional healing. Grief is a spontaneous response to loss and the normal way to adjust to endings and change [32].

Grief often begins with the initial anticipation of loss [33]. Grievers may progress through various phases of grief [32,34]. Shortly after the loss, clients may experience numbness, which may be accompanied by confusion, shock, anger, or denial. This may be followed by a period of searching or yearning for the loved one to return. The next phase may be a period of disorganization associated with strong emotions of despair and difficulty with day-to-day functions. Finally, the bereaved person begins to accept the reality of the loss and to integrate this loss into his or her current life.

An adaptive grief process may last for days, weeks, months, or even years, depending on the significance of the loss. If grief progresses in an adaptive manner, manifestations lessen in intensity over time [33]. Indicators of complicated grief include a prolonged period of grieving, intense responses, and interference with physical or emotional well-being [35,36]. Clients displaying a complicated grief reaction may benefit from referral to a mental health professional sensitive to the needs of those grieving the death of a pet.

Is there a "right" way to grieve? The grief response is unique to each individual. Therefore, there is no "best" way to grieve. The intensity of each person's grief response is based on multiple unique factors, such as the nature of the loss; the circumstances surrounding the loss; and the griever's age, gender, cultural background, and emotional status as well as the availability of emotional support before, during, and after loss [37]. When the expression of grief is restricted, the healing period for recovery is prolonged. When grief is freely expressed, the healing time for recovery from loss is greatly reduced [33]. Veterinarians can best help clients to cope with the death of a pet effectively by encouraging open expressions of grief and by empathizing with their loss [2,22].

DELIVERING BAD NEWS

Bad news has been defined as "any news that drastically and negatively alters the person's view of her or his future" [11]. A more inclusive definition of bad news is ". . .situations where there is either a feeling of no hope, a threat to a person's mental or physical well-being, a risk of upsetting an established lifestyle, or where a message is given which conveys to an individual fewer choices in his or her life" [10].

There are no strategies or methods that allow veterinarians to break bad news painlessly. Although it is difficult, veterinarians should prepare themselves for a range of client reactions that are largely unpredictable. Some clients may react with anger or blame or with overwhelming feelings of guilt, shock, disbelief, or sadness, and others may appear calm, stoic, or under control. Processing bad news differs for each individual and may require various amounts of time to deal with the news. Through effective techniques, the bad news encounter can be made less distressing for the veterinarian and the client, support long-term relationships with clients, and enhance veterinarian and client satisfaction during a challenging conversation [10–12,22,23].

One useful model for delivering bad news is the SPIKES six-step model developed by Buckman [11] and employed in many medical school curricula. This model provides a structured approach to delivering bad news, and its principles are relevant to the practice of veterinary medicine. Evidence indicates that focused educational interventions using a stepwise model and providing opportunities for practice and observation of actual behaviors as well as provision of feedback, with repetition and reinforcement throughout the curriculum, result in improved communication skills [10].

Setting

- Create an appropriate setting to ensure privacy, client and patient comfort, and lack of distractions. Allow for time, discussion at eye level, and invitation of supportive individuals. A designated clinical comfort room would be a suitable environment in which to deliver bad news.
- Identify who should be present for the conversation:

I am wondering if there are other persons who care about Max who may want to take part in this discussion.

- Take time to establish initial rapport with the client, using open-ended questions, compliments, and empathy statements:

How are you doing?
I am glad that you brought Max in, so that we could address this problem.
The last 24 hours has been really tough.

Perception

- Explore the client's perspective about the pet's illness, using open-ended questions:

What are your concerns regarding Max's condition?
What do you think is causing Max's illness?
Tell me in your own words what you understand about Max's disease.

- Determine the client's desire for information. People have different ways of coping with bad news [12]. Some cope by learning as much as they can so that they can feel in control, and others prefer not to know and cope by avoiding thinking about it. Evidence in medical communication indicates that physicians underestimate how much information patients would like to receive [38–40]. Although most patients would like more information from their doctor, a small group would like less. Therefore, the primary goal is to tailor your discussion to individual client needs:

Some clients like to know a lot about their animal's illness and others prefer the basic facts. What would you prefer?

Invitation

- Ask permission to share the information with the client:

I am wondering if it is alright with you if I discuss some of the specifics regarding Max's illness.

Knowledge

- Deliver the bad news in stages. It is recommended that bad news be delivered in stages, because it takes time for clients to realize the full magnitude of what they have been told [41].
- Provide a warning shot:

Mary, I have some difficult information to share with you regarding Max's condition [Pause].

- Give information in small easily understandable pieces. Share only one to three sentences at a time, and pause and check for the client's understanding before proceeding. Chunking and checking allows the veterinarian to tailor the discussion based on the amount and type of information desired by the client, resulting in enhanced recall of information and engendering a shared understanding [42]:

The cancer has spread to Max's lungs. This will continue to make it very hard for Max to breathe and will eventually cause his death [Pause].

- Ask for the client's permission to continue to disclose the details of the medical condition:

Would you like me to tell you more about Max's condition now, or would you like to talk later, perhaps at another time when you can bring a friend along with you?

- Check for the client's understanding, using open-ended questions:

What questions do you have at this point?
What additional information may be helpful to you?
Tell me how you understand the choices for Max's care.
What do you think are the most important points to present to your family?

- Avoid use of technical jargon and define medical terms.
- Use supplemental tools, such as written materials or audiotape recordings. Studies indicate that patients only remember approximately 50% of what their physician said [42]. Therefore, providing client information sheets or discharge instructions may help clients to recall key points after the visit. Tape recordings allow clients to listen to the information again when they are in a more relaxed familiar environment or to share with family members [43].

Empathize

- Throughout the conversation, acknowledge, validate, and normalize the client's emotional responses.
- Use silence and empathetic statements, and display compassionate and caring nonverbal cues (ie, sit close to the client; mirror facial expressions; use a gentle, calm, and caring tone of voice; use a slow pace of speech; lean forward; use touch). Practitioners sometimes struggle with finding the right words to say; however, being a caring presence through silence and nonverbal communication can provide just as much comfort to the client:

I'm right here for you. Take your time.
I can imagine how hard this is for you to talk about. This news is overwhelming.
This is a lot of information to absorb, and it came unexpectedly.
It seems to me like you want to make the decision in Max's best interest.

Summary and Strategy

- Summarize what has been discussed.
- Negotiate a plan for treatment or follow-up.

- Identify client support systems:

I am wondering who in your life will support you in making decisions regarding Max's care.

- Provide information on support services (ie, grief counseling, support groups).

EUTHANASIA DECISION MAKING

The term *euthanasia* is derived from the Greek *eu* meaning "good" and *thanatos* meaning "death" [44]. Positive words like humane, gift, and painless are associated with companion animal euthanasia; yet, as a medical procedure, euthanasia is the purposeful act of terminating life [45]. Given the deep emotional relationships that many people share with their pets, discussing euthanasia is stressful for pet owners and veterinary professionals [46].

In veterinary medicine, the primary goal of end-of-life decision making is ensuring quality of life during the treatment or palliative care phase and, ultimately, a peaceful timely death for a terminally ill or injured patient. Clinical experience demonstrates that this process can be heavily influenced by many factors, including the pet's level of pain, clinical signs, diagnosis, prognosis, and response to treatment or palliative care options; the owner's psychoemotional resilience and ability to provide care for the animal; and the ability of those involved in the decision-making process to arrive at a consensus.

Discussing euthanasia is challenging for clients and veterinarians [2,8,45]. Veterinarians often initiate and facilitate euthanasia discussions when they know that death is near. End-of-life discussions clarify the client's wishes regarding the pet's death, help to minimize regrets about how the pet's death was handled, and allow the client to cope with the death of the pet. Once again, the SPIKES six-step model [11,47] provides a useful structure on how to conduct a euthanasia decision-making conversation with a client.

Setting

- Create an appropriate setting (see previous guidelines).
- Establish initial rapport, using empathy statements, open-ended questions, and compliments:

It seems like you have been on a roller coaster for the last few months. How are you doing? How do you feel Max is doing?
This has been a tough time for both you and Max.

Perception

- Establish what the client knows about the pet's illness (see previous guidelines).
- Understand the client's perspective and values on end-of-life care, using open-ended questions:

How do you think we should balance treating Max's cancer and ensuring quality of life [48]?

What are your hopes for Max? What are your fears for Max [48]?
What makes life worth living for Max [48]?
Under what circumstances would life not be worth living for Max [48]?
What do you think Max's quality of life is like now [48]?

- Ask about the client's previous experiences with euthanasia, using open-ended inquiry:

I am wondering whether you have had previous experiences with making a euthanasia decision. What factors came in to play in making that decision?
I am wondering whether you have been present at a euthanasia procedure in the past. Tell me about that situation.

- Explore religious or spiritual beliefs that may have an impact on a euthanasia decision, using open-ended inquiry:

Some clients have religious or spiritual beliefs that guide the euthanasia decision. I am interested in how these beliefs might guide your decision-making process.

Invitation

- Obtain the client's permission to discuss euthanasia. The veterinarian's role is vital in facilitating these discussions, including giving permission for clients to consider euthanasia as an option, acknowledging the difficulty in making such a decision, and allowing clients to express their feelings and desires openly [49]. Using words that reflect partnership (ie, "we," "be there") comforts the client in knowing that he or she is not alone in making this decision:

I am wondering whether it would be alright with you if we took a few minutes to discuss the option of euthanasia.
We can hope for the best in Max's care, and we also need to plan for the future so that we can ensure Max's quality of life.
No matter what the road holds ahead, I am going to be there for you and Max [50].

Knowledge

- Provide a warning shot:

This is one of the most difficult decisions a client faces in caring for his or her pet.
Making this decision on Max's behalf is not easy. I wonder if it sometimes feels overwhelming [50]?

- Provide accurate and detailed information about the animal's condition:

Max is probably feeling like you do when you have a bad flu. It probably hurts just to move, and it is difficult for him to get comfortable. His body temperature is high, and he is having difficulty breathing [Pause] [22].

Because I haven't seen Max for 3 weeks, his decline seems quite dramatic to me. He has lost a great deal of weight and muscle tone and seems far less responsive. I believe he is experiencing quite a bit of pain. Although I can give him more medication for his pain, his disease will continue to cause him to suffer [Pause] [22].

- Give information in small easily understandable pieces, pause, and check the client's understanding before proceeding. Some clients need time to accept the decision to euthanize their pet; therefore, the euthanasia decision-making discussion may extend over several visits.
- Provide instructions on how to monitor the pet's condition. Clients often wonder out loud how they are going to know when the time is right for euthanasia. Anticipating death and knowing that it is near can be intimidating, overwhelming, and anxiety provoking. Therefore, having solid concrete information about what to watch for and what to do may make the decisions feel more manageable:

Mary, things to watch for in Max are a decrease in his appetite and interest in drinking water; reduced activity level; difficulty in breathing, such as panting or increased effort; and a lack of interest or responsiveness to you and his daily activities.

- Ask for the client's permission to continue to disclose the details of the euthanasia procedure:

I am wondering if it would be alright with you if I were to walk you through the euthanasia procedure we use at our clinic.

There are a few options and decisions in relation to the euthanasia procedure and body care, and I am wondering if you would like to discuss them now.

- Avoid use of technical jargon and define medical terms.
- Avoid the phrase "nothing more can be done," and reframe using the phrases "supportive care" or "palliative care":

We will provide supportive care to Max to make his life as comfortable as possible.

Empathize

- Throughout the conversation acknowledge, validate, and normalize the client's emotional responses.
- Use silence and empathetic statements and display compassionate and caring nonverbal cues:

I want you to know that I fully support your decision and will do my best to honor your wishes for Max [49].

You have taken such good care of Max throughout his illness. I can tell how much you love him [50].

It's quite common for clients in your situation to have a hard time making these decisions. It feels like an enormous responsibility [50].

Of course, talking about this makes you feel sad. It would not be normal if it didn't [50].

Summary
- Summarize what has been discussed.
- Negotiate a plan for treatment or follow-up.
- Identify client support systems.
- Provide information on support services (ie, grief counseling, pet loss support hotlines and groups).

IMPLEMENTATION
The Practice Culture
The practice culture influences whether end-of-life communication is valued by the veterinary team and thereby addressed or overlooked [9]. Role modeling, acknowledgment of the death, and interactions with team members have been identified as instrumental factors in skill acquisition and development of healthful coping mechanisms [7]. Practice leaders are role models not only in demonstrating skills but in displaying attitudes. Taking time to reflect on challenging conversations, the death of patients, and expressing your emotions may have an impact how your team does this.

Communication Rounds
Conducting regular communication debriefing rounds is one mechanism by which compassion, the ability to cope with losses, and skill development can be enhanced. Unlike traditional clinical rounds, the purpose of communication rounds is to reflect on interactions with clients and team members. Such rounds are conducted with the Oncology Service at Colorado State University on a weekly basis and are regularly attended by students, interns, residents, technicians, and clinicians, all of whom actively contribute to the discussion. Such dialogue fosters open communication, expression of emotion, elicitation of concerns, provision of support for team members, and acquisition of skills. The goal of these conversations is the ongoing development of a safe and supportive environment within the team. These conversations assist professionals in finding an appropriate balance between the perceived need for objectivity and the natural tendency to identify and relate to clients and patients and to respond emotionally to losses.

Facilitation
To ensure safety and supportiveness as well as to provide structure to the discussion, it is important to identify a skilled facilitator. Someone within the practice team may possess the necessary skills, or you could partner with a professional in mediation or mental health counseling to lead these rounds.

A good facilitator is someone who is an esteemed, respected, empathetic, and trusted team member who possesses strong communication skills. The role of the facilitator is primarily to ask questions, foster discussion, elicit contributions from the group, and summarize key points. Although facilitators offer input and make suggestions, it is often more meaningful to do so after obtaining input from the team. An effective facilitator uses a collaborative approach, recognizing the importance of collective expertise, compared with a paternalistic approach, in which the facilitator directs the group as the sole expert. A model is provided here, including example scripts for setting the stage for communication rounds and examples of guiding questions that can be used by a skilled facilitator.

Example Script: Communication Rounds

Setting the stage

Facilitator:

> The purpose of these rounds is to set aside time each week to reflect on our interactions with clients and with team members. This is an opportunity to discuss communication situations that you found challenging for any reason or to present a communication scenario that you thought was successful. I am wondering whether anyone had a client interaction from the past week that they would like to share.

Fostering discussion

Facilitator guiding questions include the following:

- Tell us what happened.
- What was that like for you?
- What do you attribute to the success or difficulty of this interaction?
- What impact has this situation had on the team?
- What effect did this interaction have on the client?
- How might you approach this situation differently next time around?
- What suggestions do you have?
- What has worked well for you in the past?
- What other experiences can you draw from?
- How has this experience influenced how you plan to work with clients in the future?
- What changes might we implement based on this experience?
- What do you do to care for yourself when you are feeling stressed?

SUMMARY

Skillful facilitation of end-of-life discussions is part of every veterinarian's ethical responsibility as stated in The Veterinarian's Oath [29]. Given the expectations of the profession and clients and the resultant impact of end-of-life conversations on pet owners and the veterinary team, compassionate communication is considered to be a core clinical skill and an integral part of the job of the veterinary team [2,3,28]. Through use of effective techniques, end-of-life discussions can be made less distressing for the veterinarian and the client, maintaining long-term relationships with clients and enhancing veterinarian and client satisfaction [10–12,22,23]. These skills can be taught and are a series of learned skills. Even more importantly, these skills can be modeled and foster a culture that supports clients and their pets and enhances satisfaction of the veterinary team.

ADDITIONAL RESOURCES

For more specific information on communication skills, such as nonverbal communication, open-ended questions, reflective listening, and empathy statements, the reader should consult the recent article by Shaw [51].

For more complete and applied information regarding client-present euthanasia discussions and procedures, the reader should consult the book by Lagoni and colleagues [3] on the human-animal bond and grief.

For veterinary team and client resources on pet loss and grief, the reader should consult the web sites of the Argus Institute (www.argusinstitute.colostate. edu) [52] and www.PetPeopleHelp.com [53].

References

[1] Brown JP, Silverman JD. The current and future market for veterinarians and veterinary medical services in the United States. J Am Vet Med Assoc 1999;215:161–83.
[2] Adams CL, Bonnett BN, Meek AH. Predictors of owner response to companion animal death in 177 clients from 14 practices in Ontario. J Am Vet Med Assoc 2000;217:1303–9.
[3] Lagoni L, Butler C, Hetts S. The human-animal bond and grief. Philadelphia: WB Saunders; 1994.
[4] Blackwell MJ. The 2001 Inverson Bell Symposium Keynote Address: beyond philosophical differences: the future training of veterinarians. J Vet Med Educ 2001;28:148–52.
[5] Williams S, Mills JN. Understanding and responding to grief in companion animal practice. Aust Vet Pract 2000;30:55–62.
[6] Hart L, Hart B. Grief and stress from so many animal deaths. Companion Anim Pract 1987;1:20–1.
[7] Ratanawongsa N, Teherani A, Hauer KE. Third-year medical students' experiences with dying patients during the internal medicine clerkship: a qualitative study of the informal curriculum. Acad Med 2005;80(7):641–7.
[8] Mannette CS. A reflection on the ways veterinarians cope with the death, euthanasia and slaughter of animals. JAMA 2004;225:34–8.
[9] Gorman TE, Ahern SP, Wiseman J, et al. Residents' end-of-life decision making with adult hospitalized patients: a review of the literature. Acad Med 2005;80(7):622–33.
[10] Rosenbaum ME, Ferguson KJ, Lobas JG. Teaching medical students and residents skills for delivering bad news: a review of strategies. Acad Med 2004;79(2):107–17.
[11] Buckman R. How to break bad news. Baltimore (MD): The Johns Hopkins University Press; 1992.
[12] Girgis A, Sanson-Fisher RW. Breaking bad news: current best advise for clinicians. Behav Med 1998;24(2):53–60.
[13] Tinga CE, Adams CL, Bonnett BN, et al. Survey of veterinary technical and professional skills in students and recent graduates of a veterinary college. J Am Vet Med Assoc 2001;219:924–31.
[14] Eyre P. Professing change. J Vet Med Educ 2001;28:3–9.
[15] King LJ. It was the best of times, it was the worst of times. J Vet Med Educ 2000;217:996–8.

[16] Chadderdon LM, King LJ, Lloyd JW. The skills, knowledge, aptitudes and attitudes of successful veterinarians: a summary of presentations to the NCVEI subgroup (Brook Lodge, Augusta, Michigan, December 4–6, 2000). J Vet Med Educ 2001;28:28–30.

[17] Bristol DG. Using alumni research to assess a veterinary curriculum and alumni employment and reward pattern. J Vet Med Educ 2002;29:20–7.

[18] Heath TJ, Mills JN. Criteria used by employers to select new graduate employees. Vet J 2000;78:312–6.

[19] Butler C, William S, Koll S. Perceptions of fourth-year veterinary students regarding emotional support of clients in veterinary practice in the veterinary college curriculum. J Am Vet Med Assoc 2002;221:360–3.

[20] Williams S, Butler C, Sontag M. Perceptions of fourth-year veterinary students about the human-animal bond in veterinary practice and in veterinary college curricula. J Am Vet Med Assoc 1999;215:1428–32.

[21] Adams CL, Conlon PD. Professional and veterinary competencies: addressing human relations and the human animal bond in veterinary medicine. J Vet Med Educ 2004;31:66–71.

[22] Antelyes J. Difficult clients in the next decade. J Am Vet Med Assoc 1991;198:550–2.

[23] Antelyes J. Client hopes, client expectations. J Am Vet Med Assoc 1990;197:1596–7.

[24] Roberts CS, Cox CE, Reintgen DS. Influence of physician communication on newly diagnosed breast patients' psychologic adjustment and decision-making. Cancer 1994;74: 336–41.

[25] Cameron C. Patient compliance: recognition of factors involved and suggestions for promoting compliance with therapeutic regimens. J Adv Nurs 1996;24:244–50.

[26] Safron DG, Taira DA, Rogers WH. Linking primary care performance to outcomes of care. J Fam Pract 1998;47:213–20.

[27] Ptacek JT, Ptacek JJ. Patients' perceptions of receiving bad news about cancer. J Clin Oncol 2001;19:4160–4.

[28] Martin F, Ruby KL, Deking TM, et al. Factors associated with client, staff, and student satisfaction regarding small animal euthanasia procedures at a veterinary teaching hospital. J Am Vet Med Assoc 2004;224:1774–9.

[29] American Veterinary Medical Association. The veterinarian's oath, adopted by the American Veterinary Medical Association in 1999, reaffirmed 2004. In: American Veterinary Medical Association directory. Schaumburg (IL): American Veterinary Medical Association; 2006.

[30] Kurtz SM, Silverman J, Draper J. Teaching and learning communication skills in medicine. Abingdon (UK): Radcliffe Medical Press; 2005.

[31] Lagoni L. The practical guide to client grief. Lakewood (CO): American Animal Hospital Association Press; 1997.

[32] Kubler-Ross E. On death and dying. New York: Collier Books/Macmillan; 1969.

[33] Rando T. Grief, dying, and death: Clinical interventions for caregivers. Champaign (IL): Research Press; 1984.

[34] Worden JW. Grief counseling and grief therapy: a handbook for the mental health practitioner. New York: Springer Publishing Company; 1982.

[35] Glass RM. Is grief a disease? Sometimes. JAMA 2005;293(21):2658–60.

[36] Shear K, Frank E, Houck PR, et al. Treatment of complicated grief: a randomized controlled trial. JAMA 2005;293(21):2601–8.

[37] Cook ASOK. Dying and grieving: lifespan and family perspectives. New York: Holt, Rinehart and Winston; 1997.

[38] Waitzin H. Doctor-patient communication: clinical implication of social scientific research. JAMA 1984;252:2441–6.

[39] Levinson W, Kao A, Kuby A, et al. Not all patients want to participate in decision making: a national study of public preferences. J Gen Intern Med 2005;20:531–5.

[40] Epstein RA, Alper BS, Quill TE. Communicating evidence for participatory decision making. JAMA 2004;291:2359–66.

[41] Slaikeu KAN. Crisis intervention: a handbook for practice and research. Boston: Slaikeu, Allyn and Bacon; 1984.

[42] Silverman J, Kurtz SA, Draper J. Skills for communicating with patients. Abingdon (UK): Radcliffe Medical Press; 2005.

[43] McConnell D, Butow PN, Tattersall MHN. Audiotapes and letters to patients: the practice and views of oncologists, surgeons and general practitioners. Br J Cancer 1999;79: 1782–8.

[44] Fogle B. Interrelations between people and pets. Springfield (IL): Charles C Thomas; 1981.

[45] McMillan FD. Rethinking euthanasia: death as an unintentional outcome. J Am Vet Med Assoc 2001;219:1204–6.

[46] Rollin BE. Euthanasia and quality of life. J Am Vet Med Assoc 2006;228:1014–6.

[47] von Gunten CF, Ferris FD, Emmanuel LL. Ensuring competency in end-of-life care: communication and relational skills. JAMA 2000;284(23):3051–7.

[48] Quill T. Imitating end-of-life discussions with seriously ill patients: addressing the "elephant in the room." JAMA 2006;284(19):2502–7.

[49] Weissman DE. Decision making at a time of crisis near the end of life. JAMA 2004;292(14): 1738–43.

[50] Tulsky JA. Beyond advance directives: importance of communication skills at the end of life. JAMA 2005;294(3):359–65.

[51] Shaw JR. Four core communication skills of highly effective practitioners. Vet Clin North Am Small Anim Pract 2006;36:385–96.

[52] Argus Institute. Colorado State University, Fort Collins, CO. Available at: www.argusinstitute. colostate.edu.

[53] www.petpeoplehelp.com. Fort Collins, Co. Available at: www.petpeoplehelp.com.

Vet Clin Small Anim 37 (2007) 109–121

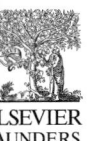

VETERINARY CLINICS
SMALL ANIMAL PRACTICE

LSEVIER
AUNDERS

Communication in the Veterinary Emergency Setting

Shane W. Bateman, DVM, DVSc

Small Animal Care and Wellness Section, Department of Veterinary Clinical Sciences,
The Ohio State University, 601 Vernon L. Tharp Street, Columbus, OH 43210-1089, USA

S uccessful communication in an emergency setting presents unique challenges to the veterinary care team and the families seeking treatment for their animal companion. Families in the emergency setting may find themselves in a strange environment facing long waiting times, interacting with multiple professionals with whom they have had no previous relationship, and, often, under circumstances that maximally challenge their coping resources. The cost of emergency services is frequently an additional source of conflict for families. Further, the severity of the medical conditions that are commonly encountered in emergency practice necessitates frequent "bad news" and "end-of-life discussions." Communication between emergency veterinary care teams and families is thus inevitably complicated by the accompanying emotional content that can be significant and potentially volatile.

Veterinary emergency medicine care teams are also faced with multiple challenges. They contend with long and undesirable working hours, recurring medical crises requiring swift and skilled responses, frequent emotionally charged interactions with clients and their families, and uncertainty of when the next crisis is likely to present or when multiple crises are likely to take place simultaneously and overwhelm the available resources of the medical team. Frequently, noise, lack of privacy, and potential for interruptions can all have a significant impact on the medical team's ability to communicate effectively with families. The medical team is also challenged by the underlying premise of emergency medicine, which is to stabilize the patient and then transfer the patient to another care team that is responsible for managing the next phase of treatment. Conflict frequently arises within the hospital as teams attempt to transfer care of patients skillfully.

The constant variety of patients and medical situations as well as the inherent challenges posed by such variety is undeniably an attraction for veterinarians who choose a career in emergency and critical care medicine. The high-pressure environment that requires quick and decisive action is alluring to "adrenaline junkies" and undoubtedly plays a role in the career choice of

E-mail address: bateman.36@osu.edu

0195-5616/07/$ – see front matter
doi:10.1016/j.cvsm.2006.09.005

the medical team and preferred communication style [1]. Medical professionals adept at managing medical crises are successful because of advanced skills in swift and calculated decision making and their ability to communicate quickly and decisively to others within medical teams. Communication that is rapid, direct, and steeped in objective medical words or jargon may be successfully used and preferred within the medical team. This preferred communication style, if used with many families, might contribute further challenges to already difficult communication situations. Therefore, to be successful, emergency medical professionals must be able to adapt their communication styles to meet the needs of many types of families and situations.

Just as the variety of conditions in emergency medicine is endless, so, too, are the principles of communication that might be applied to the emergency situation. The parameters of this article confine the discussion to consideration of the following: the elements of obtaining informed consent in a medical crisis and the components of breaking bad news to a family. Equally important to emergency communication are discussions involving talking to clients about finances, end-of-life, and euthanasia as well as approaches for attending to difficult clients or difficult situations. Fortunately, these topics are skillfully covered elsewhere in this issue.

IMPORTANT CONSIDERATIONS

"Time is limited in the emergency department. Effective communication, however, is not a function of time but rather one of skill" [2]. Perhaps the biggest barrier for emergency veterinary care teams to overcome is the commonly held belief that they simply do not have time to communicate more effectively—the perception that good communication somehow requires a lot of time. Rather, when viewed in a more comprehensive way, poor communication may actually result in investment of more time because of inappropriate diagnostic evaluations, interpersonal conflicts, repeat visits, and poor adherence.

Second, emergency veterinary care teams often care for a diverse client population. To be successful, veterinary professionals responsible for communicating with clients must be sensitive to cultural differences. They should be alert to the possibility that individual words may carry distinct meanings in different regional dialects of the same language. Further, there is the potential for two-way prejudice (veterinarian versus client and client versus veterinarian) based on race, gender, ethnicity, age, sexual orientation, religious or spiritual beliefs, social status, economic status, or literacy level. Conflict in these situations is nearly always communicated nonverbally; thus, veterinarians should be vigilant in observing any evidence of client discomfort or the possibility of being misunderstood. Such potential conflicts are best handled with open-ended questioning, reflective listening, and appropriate expressions of empathy, such as the following:

> Mrs. Garcia, I'm sensing that you are feeling uncertain about what I've told you. I'm wondering if our cultural differences might be playing a role. I want to help your family in the best way that I can; can you help me to

understand what meaning this might have for you? Can you help me to see this situation through your eyes?

OBTAINING INFORMED CONSENT

Obtaining informed consent from clients is a crucial element of ethical and professional communication in veterinary medicine. In nonurgent situations, obtaining informed consent requires the veterinarian to discuss with the client the clinical issues, the alternatives to the proposed diagnostic or therapeutic intervention (in addition to the benefits and risks of each option), and the possible adverse effects and long-term care associated with each option [3]. In addition to the standard "clinical" elements of this conversation, the veterinarian should attempt to assess the client's preferences for and understanding of the choices before him or her. This can typically be accomplished with such statements as the following:

> What is your understanding of Max's condition and the decision(s) you are facing?
> What are you thinking about regarding Max's condition?
> Tell me what factors might affect this decision for you.

Inclusion of all these elements when obtaining informed consent can help to establish and foster a shared decision-making communication model that is relationship centered.

The emergency setting can place many constraints on the process of obtaining informed consent. Most often, the urgency of a situation necessitates that this must be abbreviated. In such situations, shared decision making may not be possible for several reasons. Often, there simply is not sufficient time to establish rapport and trust with a client or family to consider shared decision making. In fact, clients may be angered by attempts to connect with them when they perceive that their companion needs the veterinarian's attention and skill more than they do. In addition, the animal may have many injuries or a complicated medical condition that cannot easily be explained in a short time frame.

Clients may also be so overwhelmed by their emotional response to the situation that they are unable to make informed decisions. In such situations, the veterinarian may adapt his or her communication style to a caretaker or guardian role. In other words, the veterinarian, as the trained medical professional, provides only the information that is perceived to be required and asks for the client's trust and approval of a medical plan that is outlined as quickly as possible. In such situations, the veterinarian may briefly inform the client of his or her companion's medical condition and important life-saving therapies that constitute the highest standard of care that can be reasonably offered. If possible, this conversation should include a realistic estimate of the likelihood of success or failure associated with treatment, the probable long-term outcome from the medical condition, and an estimate of cost associated with the immediate medical plan. If the patient is badly injured or the treatment is likely to be extremely costly, humane euthanasia should be offered as an option for consideration. So as not to influence the client's decision unduly, it is important to present the options with as little bias as possible and to communicate to the client that you are going to support his or her decision. These statements may be followed by a closed-ended question seeking the client's permission for a course of action.

An example might be the following:

> Mrs. Jones? I'm Dr. Smith. How are you holding up? [Pause for response.] I've just examined Sadie, and I'm sorry to tell you that she's been badly injured by the car that hit her. It appears that she has severe internal injuries in addition to several broken bones. We've started an intravenous line and are trying to stop the bleeding. As soon as it is safe to do so, I will give her medication to control her pain. I think we'll have to put a tube into her chest to help stabilize her collapsed lungs, and she may require a blood transfusion. We'll do everything we can to try and stabilize her condition. It's too early to know if we're going to be successful. This is, no doubt, lots of information for you to take in at once. I promise to keep you up to date on any major changes in her condition. It's also important that we discuss the estimated costs for Sadie's care; would that be okay? [Pause for response.] We might spend up to $750 while we are trying to stabilize her and determine the extent of her injuries. If we are successful, I know from the extent of her injuries that you'll be most likely be faced with total costs that may easily go above $3000. It is important for you to know that I'm still hopeful that we can save Sadie. I also think that humane euthanasia would be a responsible and reasonable decision for many families. Please know that I'd support any decision you might make. I'm sorry that I'm giving you so much information so quickly. I don't have much time to spend with you, but I can answer one or two questions. How would you like to proceed?

DELIVERING BAD, SAD, OR UNWELCOME NEWS

Some of the most distressing experiences for medical professionals are often those surrounding the delivery of bad news. Bad news has been defined as "situations where there is a feeling of no hope, a threat to a person's mental or physical well-being, a risk of upsetting an established lifestyle, or where a message is given which conveys to an individual fewer choices in their life" [4]. Veterinarians report experiencing significant anxiety and stress before, during, and after such types of communication [5]. Such encounters contain raw emotional content that can often feel overwhelming for all parties involved. The emotional exchanges between clients and veterinarians in such situations, when viewed empathetically, are often humanizing experiences. Many are landmark moments in a career, when the patient becomes the healer or the teacher becomes the learner. They can be pivotal moments that leave indelible impressions and lessons for a lifetime. The unique coping responses that clients (and veterinarians) have learned or acquired over time to deal with delivery of such news are often viewed from a jaded or self-protective perspective, however. It is often easier to make judgments about a client's emotional response to the situation or crisis when it makes us uncomfortable. The "war stories" that are frequently shared among coworkers or colleagues often share a common thread of the "craziest" or "weirdest" client or situation ever encountered. When examined more closely, such story-telling behavior speaks as loudly of our own fears and inadequacies as those of our clients. The fundamental skill needed in such situations is empathy. Digging deep within ourselves to see others who are struggling, to hear their words of confusion and pain, and to help them feel understood, all without judgment or shame, may be the most challenging and the most rewarding experiences of a career.

There is convincing work to suggest that how bad news is delivered can have a significant impact on the veterinarian-client relationship, decrease the stress for the deliverer of bad news, and improve several important outcomes from the receiver's perspective [6]. Much of the literature is grounded in empiric approaches and experiences of seasoned clinicians who have shared their experiences and pearls of wisdom.

Brewin [7] originally described three conceptual models of how clinicians might deliver the news to the receiver. Others have used his framework in discussing the "optimal" role for the deliverer of bad news. In Brewin's model, a clinician may adopt a patient-, disease-, or emotion-centered style of communication when delivering bad news. A clinician adopting the emotion-centered style is kind and sad. The clinician appears unhurried, focuses excessively on sympathy and empathy, is grave and solemn, and offers little encouragement or hope. The clinician may be motivated to deliver news in this way because of a fear of raising false hopes. The receiver of the news may focus on the nonverbal aspects of this prototypical message and might assume that the situation is worse than in actuality. The clinician delivering bad news using Brewin's disease-centered prototype couches the message in "medspeak" and is typically blunt and insensitive. The clinician's motivation may be that the message is so distressing that it really makes no difference how it is delivered. The final prototype described by Brewin is the patient-centered approach, which is described as understanding and positive. The clinician's motivation is to be truthful and deliver the message using care and flexibility depending on the expressed needs and concerns of the client. Key elements of this prototype are verifying that the client understands the message; expression of empathy and, if appropriate, encouraging the client to maintain realistic hope about the news, even if all that can be offered is symptom relief; and offering a care plan and partnership for the immediate future.

A review of human medicine literature by Ptacek and Eberhardt [4] in 1996 identified a number of useful elements suggested for use in the delivery of bad news. The authors identified select elements that represented a consensus of previous studies (Box 1). Not surprisingly, many of the elements identified fit best with the patient-centered model of delivering bad news identified previously. In addition to the recommendations of these investigators, several other protocols have been developed to assist clinicians in the delivery of bad news

Box 1: Consensus elements of delivering bad news

Physical and social setting

- Location
  - Quiet, comfortable, private
- Structure
  - Convenient time, no interruptions, enough time available to ensure no rushing
  - In person, face-to-face, make eye contact, sit close to patient, avoid physical barriers
- People
  - Support network: identify and have present at client's request

Message

- What is said
  - Preparation: give a warning shot
  - Find out what client already knows
  - Convey some measure of hope
  - Acknowledge and explore client's reaction and allow for emotional expression
  - Allow for questions
  - Summarize the discussion verbally and/or in written form, audiotape consultation

How it is said

- Emotional manner: warmth, caring, empathy, respect
- Language: simple, careful word choice, direct, no euphemisms or technical diagnostic terminology, avoid medical jargon
- Give news at person's pace, allow him or her to dictate what he or she is told

Data from Ptacek JT, Eberhardt TL. Breaking bad news—a review of the literature. J Am Med Assoc 1996;276(6):496–502.

[8–10]. Clinicians using some of these protocols have reported decreased anxiety and stress when required to deliver bad news [8,9]. Trainees have reported feeling more confident in their ability to deliver bad news after undergoing training that used protocols [9]. In summary, the literature has offered techniques that have assisted clinicians in the effective delivery of bad news. Interestingly, most of the literature emphasizes delivery of bad news from the clinician's perspective and not the client's. Clinicians have written about what they believe has been helpful to clients, yet much less has been written about the client's perspective of what elements of delivery of bad news were most helpful to them [6].

One study [11] evaluated client preferences to the three prototypical styles of bad news delivery described by Brewin [7]. Female students were recruited to watch one of three videotape clips in which a male physician delivered bad news related to breast cancer diagnosis to a female actor. The female students were instructed to place themselves in the role of the patient and to react to the physician's communication. In each clip, the physician adopted a different prototypical style. Patient preferences regarding the style of communication were extensively studied. Students viewing the patient-centered videotape rated the physician to be high in emotion, availability, expression of hope, least dominant, and most appropriate in conveying information. Students watching this videotape also reported the highest visit satisfaction and smallest increase in negative emotions. Reliance only on female volunteers to "role play" their responses rather than studying actual patients was an obvious limitation of this study. Further research on patient or client perspective on what constitutes effective delivery of bad news should address this identified gap in the literature.

Delivery of bad news by veterinarians has not been extensively studied. One survey of 62 veterinarians probed numerous hypotheses regarding the delivery of bad news [5]. The purpose of the study was to determine what factors served to reduce veterinarian anxiety or stress when delivering bad news. The results indicated that sharing bad news seems to become easier for veterinarians as they gain experience and that delivering bad news may be less stressful for veterinarians than their human physician counterparts. Veterinarians reported less stress regarding emotional reactions of their clients and, in general, thought that the techniques reported in the literature were helpful to them and to their clients.

It is also noteworthy that the intensity and timing of the stress and anxiety associated with the delivery of bad news differ for the deliverer and the receiver [4]. Typically, the person delivering the bad news experiences the most anxiety before and during the delivery; once he or she has delivered the message, the stress and anxiety abate. The receiver, conversely, does not experience the peak amplitude of stress and anxiety associated with the delivery of bad news until some later point. In some cases, this might be after the deliverer has left the room, at the reception desk, or after the client returns home. As a result, it is important that all veterinary staff be trained to handle the client's reaction skillfully. Clients may experience many complex emotional or angry responses. It is important that staff be trained not to personalize the message or to become defensive in such situations, for example:

> Mrs. Smith, I can see you are upset. Would you like to step into this exam room for a few minutes?
>
> I can see you are feeling angry. I might feel angry too, if I'd just received some bad news. Would it help to talk about what is most upsetting to you?

The Bayer Animal Health Communication Project [12] provides a an interactive training module that addresses the delivery of bad news in the veterinary context using Buckman and colleagues' five-step approach (Box 2) [13]: preparation, assessment of client knowledge and/or preferences, sharing the news,

Box 2: Bayer Animal Health Communication Project: recommendations for delivery of bad news

- Preparation
  - Review the facts—prepare what to say
  - Time and place
  - Who should be present
  - Issues likely to arise
  - How to respond
  - Review and feedback
  - Quiet place where privacy is respected
  - Pagers turned to vibrate
  - Instructions to staff for no interruptions
  - Veterinarian should be primary informer
  - It helps to review the words you plan to use and anticipate client's likely questions and reactions
- Assessment of client knowledge and preferences
  - Start where the client is (words used/avoided, nonverbal behavior)
  - Assess how much or to what degree information will be given (most clients appreciate the complete truth)
- Sharing bad news
  - Begin with forewarning
  - Use the animal's name
  - Avoid medicalese and jargon
  - Give information in small chunks
  - Keep the pace slow and allow time for client to absorb information, severity or finality
  - Client preferences may change with time
  - Use words not subject to misinterpretation, such as cancer, died, dying
- Attending to feelings
  - Be prepared for a range of reactions (eg, speechless, tearful, doubt, anger)
  - Observe for verbal/nonverbal expressions of emotion
  - Provide space for client to react
  - Supportive silence
  - Legitimize and normalize strong emotions
  - Understand that guilt is common, regardless of circumstances
  - Attend to your own nonverbal communication (eye-level, seated, eye contact, slow pace of speech, lower tone may reduce anxiety, appropriate use of touch)
- Planning and follow-through
  - Be alert for signs of distress and assess client's resources for support

- Provide message of realistic hope and support
- Be aware of you own emotional response
- Document information given

Adapted from Buckman R. How to break bad news: a guide for health care professionals. Baltimore (MD): Johns Hopkins University Press; 1992; and Buckman R, Sourkes BM, Lipkin M, et al. Strategies and skills for breaking bad news. Patient Care Canada 1996;9:33. *From* Bayer Animal Health Communication Project. Module 9: strangers in crisis: partners in care. New Haven (CT): Institute for Healthcare Communication; 2006; with permission.

attending to feelings, and enlisting the client for follow-up and planning. The preparation step is an important one, particularly for emergency clinicians. It is crucial to slow down and take a moment from a busy shift to compose your thoughts, emotions, and physical person before talking with clients.

Depending on the urgency of the situation, assessment of client knowledge and preferences may have many variations, for example:

> Before I talk about our findings, it will help me to know if you are more of a big picture or more of a detail sort of person.
> What is your understanding of Max's condition right now?
> What is your understanding of the disease called cancer?
> Mrs. Jones, it is important for you to know that while I'm still hopeful about Sid's condition, there is a good chance that Sid might die while he is under our care. It may occur suddenly without warning, or he might take a turn for the worse, and we'd be more prepared for it. If that were to happen, I'd like to understand what your family's wishes and needs would be. Would it be helpful to talk about that?

Notifying clients of an animal's death or other types of catastrophic complications may be examples of when assessment of client knowledge and/or preference may actually be skipped initially but used after the delivery of the news when assessing the family's choices about body care.

Sharing the news with the client is the next step. Depending on the complexity and nature of the bad news being presented, the information may need to be presented in smaller chunks with an adequate pause for the receiver to digest the information. Before continuing, it is helpful to check or verify understanding of the previous chunk. This technique has been described as the "chunk and check" technique, which is exemplified in the following example:

> Before we talk about the next step, which is what options can be considered to make Sally well again, do you have any questions or concerns regarding Sally's condition? What is your understanding of what I've told you?

It is also helpful to allow natural pauses to appear in the delivery of the information so as to allow the client time to absorb completely the information being provided. In addition, beginning the delivery of bad news with a fore-warning statement may assist in allowing a client to mobilize his or her own coping resources for the news to that is coming, for example:

> Mr. Brown, I've got some very difficult news to share with you. [Pause, and allow client to prepare.] As you know, Trixie's injuries were very severe. We did everything we could. I'm sorry to have to tell you that she died a few moments ago. [Pause, and allow the client to have a reaction to the news; when he or she is able to hear your next statement, continue.] We were with her when she died. I made sure she was as comfortable as I could. [Pause, and attend to client's emotional response; when appropriate to continue with news, begin assessing client preferences.] When you feel ready to discuss them, there are a few choices you'll need to make. Do you feel up to that now? First, I want you to know that you can be with Trixie and hold her or hug her; I can bring her into the room for you. [The remaining options that are pertinent to each situation, such as necropsy, type of necropsy, cremation, or burial, could be discussed here.]

Attending to the client's emotional response might be the most anxiety-provoking aspect of the experience for emergency clinicians. Learning to validate and effectively respond to the unpredictability of client expression of raw emotions can be uncomfortable depending on the veterinarian's own personal or cultural values and norms. Renowned palliative care specialist Ira Byock once remarked, "Intimacy is not a function of time" (I. Byock, personal communication, 1999). Attending skillfully and empathically to the emotional responses of clients troubled by bad news does not require that you know someone well. It simply involves learning, practicing, and being comfortable with the skills of offering empathic comments and actions that are congruent with the needs and preferences of the client. It is also important to normalize and legitimize the strong emotions that clients may be experiencing. Some examples might include the following:

> I can see how difficult this is for you.
> I hear how angry you are. It's normal to feel like that. I'd be angry too if this happened to me.
> It's understandable that you are having trouble believing that this is happening. It has all happened so quickly.
> Being angry is normal. I'm upset too that Buddy did not respond the way that we'd hoped.
> Cats sneak out of their house a lot. You didn't mean for this to happen. You got Ginger here as soon as you could. You're doing everything you can to help him. Sometimes, things just happen.

In situations when a client is facing end-of-life decisions, Ira Byock has written eloquently about four phrases that may be powerful and healing for clients to say to their pets: "Please forgive me. I forgive you. Thank you. I love you" [14]. Attending to emotional content often leads to the question of touching, or hugging a client: should I or shouldn't I? In general, if you are comfortable in offering physical gestures of reassurance, it is important and appropriate to assess the client's preference for hugging: "You look like you might use a hug. Would you like a hug?" When offering clients reassuring gestures of touch, it is important to avoid touching some areas of the body that may be threatening. The safest areas to touch are the shoulder, upper or lower arms, and the top of the hand.

The final steps include planning and follow-through. The most important elements of this step are to continue to check with the client regarding understanding of the message. Continued emotional responses are normal and often require switching back and forth from the previous step to this one. Clients who have experienced a particularly emotional response to the delivered news should be provided an opportunity to call someone who may drive them home, or at least be assessed again by hospital staff to verify that it is safe for them to drive. Equally important for clients experiencing intense emotional responses is to determine what resources are available to assist them in the future. Providing referral to support systems, such as pet-loss hotlines, pet-loss support groups, or reading material regarding pet loss, is often helpful. In addition, planning a follow-up call to the client or reassuring the client that he or she may contact you or your staff again is vital. It is normal for clients to need to ask follow-up questions and to reassure themselves that they remember all the details of what happened or what they were told. In situations other than death notification, providing a message of realistic hope is appropriate, such as the following:

> Hearing Tabitha has cancer must be hard. I'm hopeful though, that we will be able to remove all the tumor with surgery.
> This is distressing news, but at least we know what we are up against now and there is a reason to explain Sam's diarrhea.
> Ben's cancer is quite advanced, and I hear that you are not quite ready to let him go. I think there are a number of things we can try to make him more comfortable for the time he has left.

SUMMARY

Delivery of bad news, although it may be stressful, is one of the most important situations in which medical professionals communicate with clients. Clients receiving bad news that is delivered poorly are likely to experience confusion, distress, and resentment. When bad news is delivered skillfully, using some or all of the elements or strategies mentioned here, it may lead to several positive outcomes. Clients receiving skillfully delivered news experience better understanding of the medical problem and may more likely be ready and able to make decisions and accept the outcomes. Veterinarians working in emergency and critical care medicine are frequently required to deliver bad news to clients under difficult circumstances that intensify the emotional impact of the bad news, and thus may benefit from learning and using the skills and techniques identified (Appendix 1).

APPENDIX 1

As a group, discuss the situations in which you are frequently required to deliver bad news. These may be situations that you have encountered recently or in the past or situations that you have not encountered but worry you. As a group, discuss the most difficult aspect of delivering this news in that particular situation. As a group, brainstorm alternative language that you might use in your situation based on the information presented in this article. Pay particular attention to the use of open-ended inquiry, reflective listening, and empathic statements. If you are comfortable, work with a partner and role play delivery of the bad news again. Seek input from the remainder of the group. Another method may be videotaping the role play, reviewing it yourself, and then asking others for input.

Examples to get you started include the following scenarios:

1. Mrs. Jones has just presented Samantha, a 10-year-old spayed female Poodle, for further evaluation of severe respiratory distress. Samantha was previously diagnosed with severe mitral valve endocardiosis and has been hospitalized and treated twice for severe congestive heart failure. She is currently taking all the latest medications, and you are not optimistic that you can "tweak" her medications any further. She was also diagnosed with metastatic mammary carcinoma 1 month ago. You are not certain whether the current episode of respiratory distress is attributable to heart failure or neoplasia. Mrs. Jones is an elderly widow with no close family. Samantha is her lifeline, and she has told you on more than one occasion that she won't be able to face the day when Samantha "goes."

2. Mrs. Smith has just presented her 2-year-old Labrador Retriever to you after it was struck by a car. There were severe thoracic injuries; despite aggressive resuscitative efforts, the dog died within minutes of arriving at the hospital. Mrs. Smith's 10-year-old son accidentally let the dog out without a leash and has come with his Mom to the hospital.

References

[1] Sibbald B. Adrenaline junkies. Journal of the Canadian Medical Association 2003;169(9): 942–3.

[2] Knopp R, Rosenzweig S, Bernstein E, et al. Physician-patient communication in the emergency department. 1. Acad Emerg Med 1996;3(11):1065–9.

[3] Fettman MJ, Rollin BE. Modern elements of informed consent for general veterinary practitioners. J Am Vet Med Assoc 2002;221(10):1386–93.

[4] Ptacek JT, Eberhardt TL. Breaking bad news—a review of the literature. JAMA 1996;276(6): 496–502.

[5] Ptacek JT, Leonard K, McKee TL. "I've got some bad news": veterinarians' recollections of communicating bad news to clients. J Appl Soc Psychol 2004;34(2):366–90.

[6] Fallowfield L, Jenkins V. Communicating sad, bad, and difficult news in medicine. Lancet 2004;363(9405):312–9.

[7] Brewin TB. Three ways of giving bad-news. Lancet 1991;337(8751):1207–9.

[8] Baile WF, Buckman R, Lenzi R, et al. SPIKES—a six-step protocol for delivering bad news: application to the patient with cancer. Oncologist 2000;5(4):302–11.

[9] Hobgood C, Harward D, Newton K, et al. The educational intervention "Griev-ing" improves the death notification skills of residents. Acad Emerg Med 2005;12(4):296–301.

[10] Keller VF, Goldstein MG, Runkle C. Strangers in crisis: communication skills for the emergency department clinician and hospitalist. Journal of Clinical Outcomes Management 2002;9(8):439–44.

[11] Mast MS, Kindlimann A, Langewitz W. Recipients' perspective on breaking bad news: how you put it really makes a difference. Patient Educ Couns 2005;58(3):244–51.

[12] Bayer Animal Health Communication Project. Module 9: strangers in crisis: partners in care. New Haven (CT): Institute for Healthcare Communication; 2006.

[13] Buckman R, Sourkes BM, Lipkin M, et al. Strategies and skills for breaking bad news. Patient Care Canada 1996;9(2):33–40.

[14] Byock I. The four things that matter most: a book about living. New York: Free Press; 2004.

Vet Clin Small Anim 37 (2007) 123–134

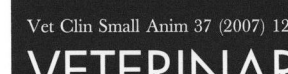

VETERINARY CLINICS
SMALL ANIMAL PRACTICE

Compassion Fatigue and the Veterinary Health Team

Susan P. Cohen, DSW

The Animal Medical Center, 510 East 62nd Street, New York, NY 10021, USA

I t has been a busy day in the clinic: one young dog hit by a car, the euthanasia of a 17-year-old cat whose family started with you when you first opened your practice, and a technician who comes in late again because she sleeps through her alarm. You wish you had her problem; you lie awake for hours staring at the ceiling and thinking about your cases. When you do fall asleep, you dream that goblins have sneaked into your operating suite and are contaminating all the equipment. You feel that no one else at work cares as much as you do. Your family does not understand, so you keep your problems to yourself. You stay so late at work that you only see your kids on weekends, and, even then, you do not have the energy to watch them at judo practice. The truth is that you would rather lock yourself in the computer room with a couple of beers.

Does this sound familiar? Are you worried about yourself? How about that sleepy technician? If so, you are wise to be concerned. You have just listed classic signs of compassion fatigue: sleep disturbance, withdrawal, hypervigilance, and self-medication (those beers).

This article summarizes the current literature about compassion fatigue, explores signs and symptoms, and suggests ways to prevent or overcome the worst parts. The article covers the history of the concept, its connection with burnout, medical and psychologic risk factors, and methods for coping.

People who choose to be veterinarians, technicians, and shelter workers usually do so, because they want to care for animals, however they often fail to include themselves in the caregiving. That failure undermines the rationale for an animal-oriented career. How can someone care for pets unless that person is healthy?

WHAT IS COMPASSION FATIGUE?
History
The term *compassion fatigue* feels like a phrase in search of a meaning. It has been used to describe various situations, such as charitable giving, medical care, and trauma recovery. To this day, definitions overlap and wander away from each other like puppies from the nest.

E-mail address: susan.cohen@amcny.org

0195-5616/07/$ – see front matter
doi:10.1016/j.cvsm.2006.09.006

Charity

In the 1980s, world events led to efforts to help solve disasters through public awareness and group activities, such as the "Live Aid" concert. Potential donors who might have enthusiastically given time and money to one disaster, for example, an African drought, found that their desire to show up and give money waned as more and more calamities surfaced. Observers called this apathy "compassion fatigue," as some commentators still do [1].

Burnout

Another use of the term *compassion fatigue* came to overlap the expression *burnout*. In the 1960s and 1970s, researchers grew aware of the hazards of working in taxing conditions, where efforts were not rewarded. If a job became persistently stressful, the worker experienced both physical signs, such as fatigue, and emotional signs, such as withdrawal, a condition known as burnout. To escape burnout, employees might begin by getting to work late or procrastinating on projects. If stress levels did not improve, they might avoid others, even family members, or drink too much alcohol. Left untreated, burnout progressed from gradual withdrawal to leaving the stressful situation altogether. For example one veterinary technician at a large teaching hospital began to limit the number of euthanasias she would do in a day. After assisting in two, she would hide in the bathroom when the call went out for a third.

Compassion Fatigue as Emotional Trauma or Secondary Posttraumatic Stress Disorder

A different theoretic base for the concept of compassion fatigue arose out of the Vietnam War. After the Vietnam War, Americans found that some returning veterans experienced ongoing stress symptoms. They experienced flashbacks, were jumpy and irritable, and seemed obsessed with the war or else refused to discuss it. Some of them drank, took drugs, or descended into mental illness and homelessness.

As researchers studied this behavior, which they called posttraumatic stress disorder (PTSD), they came to believe that even those people who were indirectly exposed to trauma could be affected. Family members, counselors, and others who heard stories, watched television coverage, or provided care for traumatized individuals showed some of the same symptoms as those who had actually lived through those events. Spouses of Holocaust survivors [2], caregivers of sexual abuse survivors [3], partners of traumatized soldiers [4], and residents of towns where accidents and terrorism had claimed lives [5,6] experienced flashbacks, sleep problems, or hypervigilance, just as if they had been traumatized directly. Some observers began to describe this as secondary PTSD. In 1989, Charles Figley [7] applied the term *compassion fatigue* in connection with PTSD, and by 1995, he argued that those who helped people experiencing PTSD were at risk for "secondary traumatic stress disorder" [8].

Burnout Versus Compassion Fatigue

Although many people use the terms *burnout* and *compassion fatigue* interchangeably, they are two different concepts. Burnout stems from work stress and is associated with higher levels of cortisol, the stress hormone [9]. Health care workers have been extensively studied and report that burnout comes from high job demands with few external rewards [10] as well as from lack of personal or vacation time [11]. If workers who are subjected to urgent demands, lack of appreciation, and lack of relaxation do not correct the situation, they may withdraw emotionally before quitting altogether. People who burn out are like a match that has used up all its energy and gone cold.

As the name suggests, PTSD occurs in vulnerable people who have been exposed to a traumatic event. Although research continues, it seems that risk factors and effects are physical and mental. Unlike burnout, PTSD is associated with lower cortisol levels that are possibly attributable other hyperreactions in the body [12]. Exposure to severe stress can cause the hippocampus, the part of the brain that deals with memory and stress, to shrink. In PTSD, there is evidence from a study of identical twins that those who are most vulnerable may have had a smaller than average hippocampus even before the traumatic event [13]. Researchers believe that PTSD shows a unique biologic pattern that sets it apart from the normal stress response [14]. Little if any research has been done to confirm these changes in those with secondary PTSD.

The psychologic risks for PTSD also differ from those for burnout. Most studies agree on three factors: a preexisting psychiatric disorder, a family history of psychiatric disorders, or a prior history of trauma [15,16].

Although many scholars agree that those who care for traumatized individuals, as family or as professionals, show many of the same symptoms as the original victim; personality characteristics and degree of exposure may also come into play. Figley [17] suggests that it is enough just to be "someone who really, deeply cares." Because the veterinary health and animal welfare fields are full of people who care deeply, the risk for them to develop compassion fatigue is high.

Two other risk factors have been discussed in the literature: gender and exposure to traumatized people. Although PTSD occurs in men and women, symptoms and backgrounds may vary between the genders. One study finds that men have different symptoms. They show more hypervigilance (heightened awareness of danger), more irritability, and more alcohol use. The same study finds that women with PTSD have a different life experience than men, in that more women report a history of sexual abuse. [18]. Another risk factor may be the degree to which family members and caregivers have been exposed to traumatized individuals. A study of clergy helping victims of the attacks of September 11, 2001 found a direct correlation between hours spent at Ground Zero and compassion fatigue. The more time the clergy spent, the higher was their risk for developing compassion fatigue [19].

If burnout is like a match flaring up and then going cold, compassion fatigue is like the heroine of the Hans Christian Anderson tale, "The Red Shoes." The story is of a young girl who becomes captivated by a pair of red shoes. When she should be praying in church or taking care of her sick guardian, all she can think of is dancing in her red shoes. Finally, the shoes take over her life, forcing her to dance endlessly night and day, over meadow and hill, cut off from family and friends. Her solution to the problem is too grim to repeat, but when she is done, she can dance no more. Like the young girl in the story, caregivers can become consumed with activity. They may recognize the toll it is taking on their lives. Nevertheless, they are unable to stop, sometimes until permanent damage is done to their health and relationships.

EFFECTS OF COMPASSION FATIGUE

Signs and Symptoms

Like many problems, compassion fatigue develops slowly. By the time a person truly recognizes that something is wrong, he or she may have a host of problems, including the following:

1. Dissociation
2. Numbness
3. Isolation
4. Hypervigilance
5. Sleep problems
6. Tearfulness
7. Avoidance and/or obsession

Persistent stress is hard on the body. Animals, including human beings, have built-in mechanisms to respond to danger. Imagine you were on your way home from work and saw Godzilla charging at you. Your body would release steroid hormones, such as cortisol, and neurotransmitters, such as adrenaline. These help the other parts of the body to organize so as to combat or run away from danger, the well-known condition of "fight or flight."

People tend to handle persistent stress in one of two ways: they try to conserve energy, or they remain overcharged. One way to conserve energy is to disconnect from stressors, such as pressures at work or frightening experiences. People may be present in the flesh but not in the mind; a condition known as dissociation. Dissociation happens when people mentally separate themselves from the real world. Anyone who has gotten lost in a movie has experienced mild dissociation.

Sometimes people cope with a traumatic experience by "going away" from the event; a more extensive kind of dissociation. If the experience, such as repeated abuse, is severe and ongoing, a person can become so expert in going away that what began as a protective device becomes its own problem. The person may experience memory lapses or develop what can seem like other identities. He or she may react inappropriately to danger. For example, one man who watched his house burn down during a fire in the hills above Oakland, California cheerfully told rescuers that he was lucky to have such a great view [20].

Numbness is a different kind of disconnection. The shock of hearing bad news can make one temporarily unable to feel. Repeated psychologic blows can lead someone to turn off feelings altogether just to get through the day.

Another way that people try to conserve energy under stress is isolation. They quit seeing friends and spend their time at home with the computer instead of tucking their kids into bed. They may come to believe that because no one understands their situation anyway, there is no point in trying to discuss it.

Another set of reactions to trauma and stress involves overreaction, or staying overcharged. Hypervigilance is a heightened state of alertness to the possibility of danger. It makes people wary and anxious. Their constant state of readiness to protect themselves and their family can ultimately become exhausting. Ask any New Yorker who lived through September 11, 2001, and you will likely find someone who anxiously checked the sky whenever a plane seemed to be flying too low for months afterward.

Sleep problems are a sign of depression and of stress. Someone may sleep far more than usual or may have difficulty in falling or staying asleep. Sleeplessness can leave the sufferer open to illness, drowsiness, and other troubles that can make the underlying stress even worse.

Many people experiencing compassion fatigue report crying more often. Sometimes, they cry over something specific, such as a pet they have cared for that dies. Other times, they cry from a feeling of helplessness to fix everything at their job or to explain their situation to friends and family. Often, they find themselves tearful for no reason that they can identify. It catches them off guard when they are taking their morning shower or driving home after another endless day at work.

The last group of mechanisms for coping with compassion fatigue is a pair of opposites: obsession and avoidance. Some people who have been through a terrible experience or a chronically distressing one focus on it over any other interest. They collect newspaper clippings, watch every television program, and discuss the event or issue endlessly. Other people handle their experience by avoiding any exposure. This technique causes them to shun anything that might be remotely related to the source of their distress, which, like isolation, can narrow their lives and cut them off from others.

COMPASSION FATIGUE AND THE ANIMAL HEALTH AND WELFARE TEAM

Like other human beings, members of the animal health and welfare professions are vulnerable to compassion fatigue. In addition, veterinarians, technicians, and other animal care workers have special stressors that put them at risk. Some stressors and risks are shared, and some are particular to a job.

Generally, all animal care workers share a love of pets and wildlife. Many workers have fond feelings for livestock and working animals. They go into their fields to help animals live a healthier and happier life. In many cases, they make a financial sacrifice to do this work. Dr. G. is an example. A brilliant student, he was accepted at several medical schools but chose a career in veterinary medicine, where he worked for 30 years in a nonprofit institution making far less than he would have in human health care.

Some of the difficulties faced by different professions are discussed in the next sections.

Veterinarians

Veterinarians have responsibility for life and death. At any moment, doctors may find themselves confronted with a patient's blood and pain—a patient whose life depends on the doctor's skill and quick thinking. After a sudden emergency or complex procedure, many doctors fail to restore themselves. Instead of relaxing, they wear their exhaustion like a badge of honor.

As medicine has become more sophisticated, clients may request miracles that carry with them ethical dilemmas. Should the oncologist try one more protocol with little chance of success or urge the client to consider euthanasia? Should the doctor intervene when a regular client adopts out kittens that have been exposed to feline leukemia virus (FeLV) without telling the new owners?

In today's practices, high-level care and decision making are often done while dealing with clients who feel that their pet is part of the family. Depending on the doctor, this attachment may enhance the experience or make it more draining. Some veterinarians claim to have chosen their profession because they did not want to deal with human beings. The flaw, of course, is that even a herd of dairy cattle does not walk into a practice on their own. To treat patients, the veterinarian must have some skill at managing people.

Doctors who are unaware of their own needs can find themselves overtired from dealing with people. The facilitator of a workshop on personalities held at The Animal Medical Center suggested that all the doctors who had never taken the Meyers-Briggs Personality Inventory (MBTI) take a short version on-line. Among other things, this inventory tests for whether a person is an introvert or extravert. Introverts recharge by being alone, whereas extraverts get their emotional juice from being around other people. A few days later, an apparently outgoing fun-loving resident stopped the facilitator in the hall. "That workshop changed my life," he declared. "I couldn't understand why I needed to be alone for a few hours after work. I felt guilty because I didn't want to call my friends. Now I get it: I'm an introvert."

Veterinarians are selected for many of the same characteristics as doctors who treat people. Both groups are smart, and both operate independently. Both require skills for coping with death and loss. Learning to achieve appropriate emotional distance, however, can become a pernicious lack of empathy. Bellini and Shea followed 61 doctors from internship through their residency in internal medicine. The researchers tested doctors for mood changes six times and interpersonal reactions five times. Although most measures of personal distress peaked during the internship before returning to near baseline at the end of the residency, "empathetic concern" and some mood disturbances never recovered from their peak [21].

Other veterinarians may overcommit to clients and patients. These doctors pride themselves on their late hours and long telephone calls. No client request is too demanding. Even when coworkers express concern or point out that being late to appointments causes problems for the rest of the staff, the overcommitted doctor believes that he or she must do everything himself or herself. "You don't understand. This woman has no one else to talk to. She still feels guilty about the euthanasia. I know I am giving her an hour a week on the phone, but she needs it."

Another issue that affects veterinary staff is access to drugs. Some veterinarians and others may self-prescribe beta-blockers to calm themselves before a speech. Others experiment with whatever gets them high. Some veterinarians have even used the euthanasia solution to take their own lives (personal observation). Like any substance abuse problem, what may begin as an occasional fling for fun can become a frequent foray into the drug cabinet.

Technicians

Veterinary technicians share some of the same risks for compassion fatigue as veterinary doctors and have some risks of their own. Because law and standard practice put doctors in charge, technicians have less control over their work situation. They must do what the veterinarian wants, when the veterinarian wants it.

If the practice is large, some technicians have little client contact and can feel left out of the loop. Decisions about patient care are often made without technician input, leading to ethical dilemmas about treatment and euthanasia. Technicians medicate recumbent cats in end-stage renal failure and watch helplessly as dogs in heart failure struggle to breathe in oxygen cages. When given the opportunity to talk, technicians have said, "The doctor must be lying to those people. That dog needs to be put to sleep yesterday. He's suffering, and I didn't go to school to torture animals." In reality, the veterinarian may have given the clients all their options and recommended euthanasia, but if the clients are not ready, the staff must continue to treat the animal. If the veterinary practice does not regularly discuss cases with the whole staff, technicians can feel isolated in their devotion to patients, which is a setup for compassion fatigue.

Office Staff

It is not only those with hands-on responsibility for animals that can experience the stress that can lead to compassion fatigue. Office staff, such as receptionists and office managers, may also confront sick or dying animals rushed in by anxious owners. While veterinarians, technicians, and other health care personnel race to the treatment area to stabilize the animal, front desk staff are left to get information from clients who may be upset and angry. This staff must calm the family, comfort them, and relay messages from the doctor. What is even more challenging is that no matter how the clients treat them, staff members must remain calm and supportive.

Shelter Workers

Another group of workers whose stress can lead to compassion fatigue are those who staff animal shelters. In addition to the problems of dealing with animal emergencies and human emotions, shelter workers face the miseries of pet overpopulation. Although many who work in shelters do it because they love animals, they are forced to euthanize hundreds of healthy dogs and cats every year because there are not enough homes for them. In an article on the ethics and morality of pet euthanasia, Bernie Rollin [22] described this as moral stress. Friends and neighbors blame the human victims of this societal problem, shunning them at the grocery store and making snide comments at the neighborhood barbecue. As shelter workers find themselves overcommitted and underappreciated, some eventually grow isolated and cold or enmeshed and fanatical.

SELF-TEST

By now, the reader may recognize some of these difficulties. How can a person tell whether he or she is experiencing compassion fatigue? The following test can suggest the answer. Although this is not a validated psychologic instrument, the questions come from research findings and have proven useful in the author's teaching and clinical work.

In the last 2 weeks, have you

1. Been extremely upset or tearful because of work stress?
2. Avoided television, movies, or newspapers that remind you of scary, upsetting events?
3. Mentally taken work home because you can't stop thinking about upsetting things you have seen?
4. Had trouble sleeping or had bad dreams about work?
5. Felt that you cannot manage your life or that it feels out of control?
6. Felt cut off from family, friends, coworkers, or society in general?
7. Been unable to stop giving, even though you know you are running out of resources?
8. Kept your problems to yourself?
9. Given up activities that you enjoy?
10. Snapped at people?
11. Been easily startled?
12. Drunk more alcohol or used other mind-altering drugs, eaten more junk food, smoked more, used more sleeping aids, shopped more, or gambled more than usual?

Most test takers say "yes" to at least 1 of the 12 items. Anyone who says "yes" to more than half of the questions may be experiencing compassion fatigue. If so, it is time to take action.

WHAT TO DO ABOUT COMPASSION FATIGUE

So far this article has defined compassion fatigue, given its history and theoretic base, described its signs and symptoms, explored its risk factors for various members of the animal health care team, and provided a test to see whether it may already be doing damage. Perhaps the reader has acknowledged signs of compassion fatigue and wants to address it; maybe he or she wants to prevent it before it takes hold. In either case, try self-care first.

Self-Care
Set limits
The first step to short-circuit compassion fatigue is to set limits. Put in a normal work day and then go home. Trust coworkers to do a "good enough" job with patients, clients, and responsibilities of the practice. If the problem is too much involvement, empathize with colleagues and offer compassion to clients but also take care of yourself. People in need often have more resources than they recognize. You do not need to make up for the problems of others; help them to find their strengths.

Reconnect with the body's senses
Second, reconnect with the body's senses. When people try to conserve energy by shutting themselves off from upsetting circumstances, they often lose touch with pleasure as well. Do not gobble food while reviewing charts; before eating anything, stop to smell it. As an experiment, with eyes closed, hold that sandwich close to the face, inhale slowly, and then move the food away gradually. Notice from how far away the aroma still lingers. Take a moment to gaze at the sunset or to feel the texture of a chair. Use the computer beep that says "You have mail" as a reminder to take a deep breath. Schedule a massage to work out the kinks and learn where tension is. Connecting to the senses grounds us in the moment and makes life real.

Reconnect with people
People who experience compassion fatigue have often cut themselves off from anyone who could make demands, even their own pets and family. Reconnect with other people and with nonpatients. Talk to someone everyday about something other than work. Practice on the guy bagging groceries or the clerk at the drug store. If petting someone else's dog sets off anxiety about the ones at the shelter, try bird watching. Carve out time to ask the family about their day and then really listen. Friends, family, and acquaintances nourish the human spirit, even those of introverts.

Care for the body
Because stress takes a toll on the body, an important tool in the arsenal against compassion fatigue is caring for the body. Sleep, exercise, and nutrition restore what stress takes away. Millions of Americans fail to sleep enough to wake refreshed and feel effective all day. For people with compassion fatigue, falling asleep easily, resting long and deeply, and dreaming only sweet dreams is a distant memory. Sleep specialists recommend using the bedroom for sleep and sex only. Keeping work out of one's place of sanctuary is essential for those whose jobs can cause damage. A relaxing bath, a dark quiet room, and a regular bedtime all smooth the way to a restorative rest.

Exercise

Exercise strengthens overstressed bodies, promotes sleep, and calms anxiety. Scientists have long known that exercise raises endorphins, the feel-good chemicals of the brain. In addition, sleep specialists suggest that exercise early in the day prepares the body for sleep at night. Recent research has now confirmed that even moderate exercise is a powerful mood enhancer [23,24].

Relax, meditate

A powerful way to reduce and prevent stress is deep relaxation, combined with meditation. Relaxation can happen with just a stretch or a few deep breaths. Meditation is also a natural and easy state, where the mind is calm and focused. It can be part of other spiritual practice or something done for its own sake. There are many schools of meditation, and although it becomes the journey of a lifetime for some, most ordinary mortals with jobs and responsibilities can incorporate it into their daily lives. Some teachers recommend meditating for at least 20 minutes, but others contend that even a few seconds is better than none, especially if done several times a day [25]. To learn more, check the bookstore for approaches that seem appealing. In addition, many communities have classes in meditation and in yoga, which some people use as a moving meditation.

To get started, here is a relaxation script created by this author. Workshop attendees have found this exercise easy and useful. It deals with compassion fatigue, and the words can be read aloud into a tape recorder and played back. The script is addressed to you, the reader. Think of this as a message to yourself. Suggestions are made as if they were already true, (eg, "You enjoy work" or "You eat well"), because the unconscious responds better to that approach.

> Sit comfortably in your chair. Let the chair support you. Close your eyes, and allow yourself to relax. Notice that your breathing is becoming easier, deeper. [Pause] Now take your hands, bring them up in front of you, and imagine that you are holding a small ball of energy. The harder you squeeze this ball, the harder it resists, so that you cannot change its shape. Keep squeezing. As you squeeze, tell yourself that you are going deeper inside yourself. Now let go of everything suddenly, and feel yourself relax. [Pause]
>
> Imagine that you are floating on a soft cloud. You are deeply relaxed and feeling wonderful. Enjoy the sensation of floating easily along without effort or care. [Pause]
>
> Now look around you for something on which a movie is showing. It might be a giant screen or a pool of water, something that reflects. On this screen, you see a movie of yourself. You see yourself enjoying work, being productive, helping animals and people. You also see yourself taking care of you—taking breaks, eating properly, laughing with your colleagues. [Pause]
>
> Now see yourself leaving work feeling good about yourself. Notice that the rest of your life is just as fulfilling as work. You enjoy friends, family, hobbies. You rest well, eat well, and exercise well.

Tell yourself that you always enjoy work and the rest of your life as well. You take care of yourself as well as others. You know when to quit work and leave it for another day. You feel healthy, well rested. [Pause]

In the next week you will notice something, a sign that deepens your resolve to strike a healthy balance between work and the rest of your life. Be curious about what this sign is. [Pause]

If now is a good time to stop, come back to the room and rest a moment. [Pause] When you feel ready, open your eyes.

Professional Care

Self-care is sometimes not enough to overcome compassion fatigue. Overinvolvement, its side effects, and the methods people use to cope can become destructive. Insomnia, isolation, and substance use take on a life of their own. Think of addictions. People who have them know that the activity is bad for them. They can see that their jobs are in danger, their bank accounts have dwindled, and their families are slipping away. Overinvolvement that has distorted itself into compassion fatigue can ruin lives too. Remember the girl with the red shoes who could not stop dancing?

When compassion fatigue jeopardizes the other parts of life, it is time to seek professional help. The first stop is a physician who can evaluate the physical toll this has taken and can often recommend a counselor or psychotherapist. Good therapists can come from many professions, such as social work, psychology, medicine and nursing, family counseling, or pastoral care. Another source of referrals is friends and relatives.

Therapists should be licensed and should have experience with the kinds of problems the patient wants to discuss. Specific professional degrees and practice methods are often less important to effective work than making a good connection between the patient and therapist. If possible, speak with a couple of professionals to find the best match.

SUMMARY

This article has summarized the meaning of compassion fatigue, ways to recognize it, and techniques to prevent or overcome it. Veterinarians, technicians, and shelter workers may be at particular risk because they care so deeply for animals that they often fail to care for themselves. Restoring a healthy balance between work and other parts of life takes effort, but the benefits can be enormous.

References

[1] UNICEF calls for an end to compassion fatigue over Ethiopia's dying children. Available at: http://l-newswire.com/pr34930.html. Site accessed February 26, 2006.

[2] Lev-Wiesel R, Amir M. Secondary traumatic stress, psychological distress, sharing of traumatic reminiscences, and marital quality among spouses of Holocaust child survivors. J Marital Fam Ther 2001;27:433–44.

[3] Follette VM, Polusny MM, Milbeck K. Mental health and law enforcement professionals: trauma history, psychological symptoms, and impact of providing services to child abuse survivors. Prof Psychol 1994;25:275–82.

[4] Figley CR. Strangers at home: comment on Dirkszwager, Bramsen, Ader, and van der Ploeg 2005. J Fam Psychol 2005;19:217–26.

[5] Chung MC, Farmer S, Werrett J, et al. Traumatic stress and ways of coping of community residents exposed to a train disaster. Aust NZ J Psychiatry 2001;35:528–34.

[6] Pfefferbaum B, Seale TW, McDonald NB, et al. Posttraumatic stress two years after the Oklahoma City bombing in youths geographically distant from the explosion. Psychiatry 2000;63:358–70.

[7] Figley CR. Helping traumatized families. San Francisco (CA): Jossey-Bass; 1989.

[8] Figley CR. Compassion fatigue: toward a new understanding of the costs of caring. In: Stamm BH, editor. Secondary traumatic stress: self-care issues for clinicians, researchers, and educators. Lutherville (MD): Sidran Press; 1995. p. 3–28.

[9] Melamed S, Ugarten U, Shirom A, et al. Chronic burnout, somatic arousal and elevated salivary cortisol levels. J Psychosom Res 1999;46:591–8.

[10] Bakker AB, Killmer CH, Siegrist J, et al. Effort-reward imbalance and burnout among nurses. J Adv Nurs 2000;31(4):884–91.

[11] Whippen DA, Canellos GP. Burnout syndrome in the practice of oncology: results of a random survey of 1,000 oncologists. J Clin Oncol 1991;9:1916–20.

[12] Yehuda R. Biology of posttraumatic stress disorder. J Clin Psychiatry 2001;62(Suppl 17): 41–6.

[13] Gilbertson MW, Shenton ME, et al. Smaller hippocampal volume predicts pathologic vulnerability to psychological trauma. Nat Neurosci 2002;5:1111–3.

[14] Seedat S, Stein MB. Post-traumatic stress disorder: a review of recent findings. Curr Psychiatry Rep 2001;4:288–94.

[15] Breslau N. Epidemiologic studies of trauma, posttraumatic stress disorder, and other psychiatric disorders. Can J Psychiatry 2002;47:923–9.

[16] Silverman GK, Johnson JG, Prigerson HG. Preliminary explorations of the effects of prior trauma and loss on risk for psychiatric disorders in recently widowed people. Isr J Psychiatry Relat Sci 2001;38:202–15.

[17] Gould JE. Compassion fatigue: an expert interview with Charles R. Figley, MS, PhD. Medscape Psychiatry Mental Health 2005;8. Available at: http://www.medscape.com/viewarticle/513615_print. Site accessed October 25, 2005.

[18] Green B. Post-traumatic stress disorder: symptom profiles in men and women. Curr Med Res Opin 2003;19:200–4.

[19] Flannelly KJ, Roberts SB, Weaver AJ. Correlates of compassion fatigue and burnout in chaplains and other clergy who responded to the September 11th attacks in New York City. J Pastoral Care Counsel 2005;59(3):213–24.

[20] Goleman D. Those who stay calm in disasters face psychological risk, studies say. The New York Times. April 11, 1994. p. 20.

[21] Bellini LM, Shea JA. Mood change and empathy decline persist during three years of internal medicine training. Acad Med 2005;80(2):164–7.

[22] Rollin B. Animal euthanasia and moral stress. In: Kay WJ, Cohen SP, Fudin CE, et al, editors. Euthanasia of the companion animal: the impact on pet owners, veterinarians, and society. Philadelphia: The Charles Press; 1988. p. 31–41.

[23] Bartholomew JB, Morrison D, Ciccolo JT. Effects of acute exercise on mood and well-being in patients with major depressive disorder. Med Sci Sports Exerc 2005;37(12):2032–7.

[24] Babyak M, Blumenthal JA, Herman S, et al. Exercise treatment for major depression: maintenance of therapeutic benefit at 10 months. Psychosom Med 2000;62:633–8.

[25] Harp D. The 3-minute meditator. 3rd edition. Oakland (CA): New Harbinger Publications; 1996.

Vet Clin Small Anim 37 (2007) 135–149

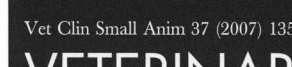

VETERINARY CLINICS
SMALL ANIMAL PRACTICE

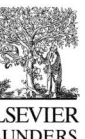

Addressing Disappointment in Veterinary Practice

Daniel O'Connell, PhD[a,b,c,*], Kathleen A. Bonvicini, MPH[a]

[a]Institute for Healthcare Communication, New Haven, CT 06511, USA
[b]Training, Coaching, and Consultation Group, 1816 1st Avenue West, Seattle, WA 98119, USA
[c]University of Washington School of Medicine, Seattle, WA, USA

THE PROBLEM

Despite the best efforts of veterinarians and the health care team, clients occasionally experience disappointment with aspects of care. Examples include perceptions of treatment they and their animal received, expectations for a specific medical outcome, and the costs of veterinary care. In the face of these disappointments, it is natural for the client to wonder about the quality of care that was provided and whether he or she was adequately informed and included in treatment decisions. Veterinary practices want clients to believe that they did the best they could under the circumstances and to conclude that the fee is reasonable for the efforts made on their behalf. This article builds on research and experience in veterinary and human medicine as well as on the broader customer service literature to address the dynamics of disappointment in small animal practices. The article goes on to offer strategies to reduce the frequency and intensity of such disappointments and to resolve them more satisfactorily when they do occur.

CHANGES IN VETERINARY MEDICINE

Like many other professions, veterinary medicine has undergone rapid change in the past several decades. For instance, there has been a significant gender reversal. Since the 1990s, more than 70% of applicants to veterinary schools in the United States have been female compared with only approximately 5% in the late 1960s [1]. In addition, the typical business of veterinary practice has shifted from an emphasis on food-producing farm animals or large animals to a focus on the "treatment of animals with no real utilitarian value other than companionship" [2]. Veterinary services showed significant growth over the past 10 years, driven by the demand for companion animal care [3]. The average dog owner in the United States spends an estimated $263 in medical expenses per dog each year and has an estimated annual expense of $113 per

*Training, Coaching, and Consultation Group, 1816 1st Avenue West, Seattle, WA 98119. E-mail address: danoconn@mindspring.com (D. O'Connell).

0195-5616/07/$ – see front matter
doi:10.1016/j.cvsm.2006.09.013

cat [4]. In fact, the pet industry as a whole has reported expansive increases in consumer expenditures in the past decade [5,6].

There are increasingly advanced diagnostic technologies available in veterinary medicine and more powerful therapeutics and surgery for the treatment of animal disease. These technical advances have created more frequent opportunities to provide specialized care. As an example, the American Veterinary Medical Association reported 7357 active specialists, an increase of 8% between 2001 and 2002 [2]. This broader range of specialties and sophisticated modalities has increased communication and decision-making challenges for pet owners and veterinarians, particularly around the care of seriously ill animals. Conditions for which euthanasia was the obvious, albeit heartbreaking choice, are now candidates for extensive treatment.

As with human medicine, increased specialization raises the question of which standard to apply when a "generalist's" care results in a disappointing medical outcome. For example, is a family practice doctor delivering babies held to the same standard of care as an obstetrician? Would the generalist veterinarian (equivalent to the primary care provider in human medical parlance) be held to the same standard as a board-certified veterinary neurologist or oncologist when he or she is caring for pets or advising pet owners in these areas? The generalist veterinarian must increasingly consider when it is appropriate to recommend referral; coordinate care with other providers; and adapt his or her practice to manage the increased communication, tracking, and follow-up obligations that come with this burgeoning of available resources (eg, laboratories, imaging, consultations).

Involving multiple providers in an animal's care also increases the possibility of the client receiving divergent opinions. Such variance may raise doubts about the quality or advisability of past and future care. Research in the malpractice area of human medicine has indicated that most lawsuits are brought about because another health care professional has suggested the possibility that malpractice has occurred [7].

Human medicine has also been criticized for physicians' reluctance to communicate directly with each other when there are diagnostic or treatment uncertainties or disagreements and an overreliance on progress notes in a medical chart in situations in which more real-time coordination is essential for patient safety [8]. Fragmentation of care and communication lapses are the most frequent contributors to adverse human medical as well as veterinary outcomes [9–12]. Trends in veterinary medicine, such as the shift from solo to group practice and the increase in the use of emergency care facilities, place additional responsibilities for transferring information, coordinating treatment plans, and clarifying roles. As a consequence, clients may not establish the kind of bond with a single veterinarian and practice setting that makes them willing to give the "benefit of the doubt" in the face of a future disappointment.

The trend toward more complex and expensive veterinary visits for companion animals has the potential for unintended consequences in the veterinary team–client relationship of a practice. Business consultants have encouraged veterinary practices to increase revenue per visit as a way to increase overall income. Clients are encouraged to bring their pets in for annual examinations, preventive care, purchasing of foods and pet care products sold in the veterinarians' offices, and such services as the implantation of identification chips [13]. Veterinarians as "trusted advocates" can become veterinarians as "small-business entrepreneurs" in clients' minds if this is not done sensitively [14].

Emerging diagnostic procedures, surgery, and therapeutics make it more likely that the last weeks and months of a pet's life could bring significant veterinary medical involvement, and thus cost, to pet owners. With 85% of small animal pet owners describing their pet as a "family member" [13], pet owners are often in a psychologically vulnerable position when they make decisions about advanced veterinary medical care. Owners' affection for and identification with their pets may drive them toward agreeing to treatment plans that may prove cumbersome, expensive, and, ultimately, unsuccessful in improving or prolonging an acceptable qualify of life. As simple a shift as the increasing use of credit cards for payment may lower the client's threshold for agreeing to care that later reveals itself to be financially imprudent. In human medicine, health insurance has provided some insulation between actual treatment expenses, payment to the provider, and cost to the consumer. Without the buffering of pet health insurance, the pet owner faces an increasingly large veterinary bill at the same time as he or she is grieving over the loss of a companion animal. Veterinarians must be ready to argue for the cessation of burdensome care in futile situations in the face of a pet owner's angst-driven inability to let go, as they enact their ethical responsibility to differentiate between their dual role as a trusted advisor and a business person who stands to profit from providing the additional services.

DISAPPOINTING OUTCOMES IN VETERINARY CARE

There is a natural tendency for pet owners to seek explanations for disappointing medical outcomes [15]. Yet, we know that in human medicine, communication problems rather than negligent medical care are the most frequent source of disappointment [16]. Many problems occur in human and veterinary medicine when there is a disparity between the outcome a client expects from a service and the actual result. For example, a client may not fully understand that individual animals have idiosyncratic responses to diagnostic tests and treatments and that the clinical presentation of an underlying condition may vary significantly from animal to animal or between testing of the same animal over time.

As a result of this biologic variability, decisions made by the veterinarian represent hypotheses that are tested by the animal's response to treatment or the progression of symptoms and signs over time. Before a stated diagnosis, other tentative diagnoses and treatment pathways may be considered and discarded. To the client, this "hypothesis testing" approach can be confused with diagnostic and treatment errors unless this process is made explicit. Even reasonable care plans have known complications and side effects that can shake clients' confidence when they do occur. Hindsight bias can make these outcomes seem more predictable, and thus preventable, than they actually were unless the client was apprised of their potential in advance [17].

Finally, there are disappointing medical outcomes that are the result of care that is later judged to have fallen below the accepted professional standard. Errors are common in human and veterinary care. Errors have been defined as the failure to complete a plan of action as intended or the use of the wrong plan to achieve the clinical aim. Breach of the standard of care is largely established by determining that similarly trained providers with the information available at that time would have recognized the error and taken a different course of action and prevented harm. Myriad interacting factors, such as attention lapses, communication failures, equipment difficulties, and knowledge deficits, may all be implicated [18]. Determining the relevant "standard of care" and evaluating the veterinarian's treatment against that standard is a central feature in determining malpractice [19,20]. In these instances, pet owners may experience even greater distress at what they conclude was the preventable suffering or loss of their animal [21]. The veterinarian is faced with the ethical, emotional, and practical challenges of sensitively communicating an accurate and potentially self-incriminatory explanation of the harm and working through the disappointment toward some resolution. As in any business, the "customer" resents being charged for a service that he or she believes is below standard; thus, it should be no surprise that receiving a bill for care with a disappointing outcome is often the event that triggers a complaint or malpractice action [22].

Because we can never eliminate adverse medical outcomes, it is in everyone's best interest for the practice team to communicate effectively with the client from the outset [14]. This includes ensuring that clients have realistic expectations and understand the uncertainties in diagnosis and treatment and conducting all interactions in such a way that the veterinary practice is given the "benefit of the doubt" about its competence, thoroughness, and effort should there be a disappointment in the process or the outcome of care.

The quality of the preexisting relationship between the client and veterinarian is a significant factor in determining how the client is likely to respond after a disappointing medical outcome. In studies of human medicine's malpractice litigants, there are differences between the way the patient and/or family and the doctor view the preexisting doctor-patient relationship. Specifically, in instances of litigation, the patient and/or family typically views the doctor-patient relationship more poorly than does the doctor [23–25]. In contrast, defense attorneys often report that patients and families are less likely to initiate a formal complaint or malpractice suit against a provider they like [26]. Beyond providing orthodox and skilled technical care, staff warmth, a focus on building and maintaining positive relationships with clients, and good customer service are among the most effective risk management tools that a practice can have [27].

A MALPRACTICE CLAIM: THE ULTIMATE DISAPPOINTMENT

A malpractice claim or a complaint to the veterinary licensing board usually indicates that a client's disappointment was inadequately or poorly resolved. We now know better how most clients want professionals to respond to perceived preventable errors by themselves or their staff [22,28,29] (Under the legal principle of "master respondeat," the practice is held legally responsible for harm caused by any of its employees.) Clients desire full explanations as part of a transparent and truthful disclosure [27]. They expect to see remorse and to receive a genuine apology. They want the veterinary practice to make changes to prevent similar harm to another animal so as to provide some assurance that something good is going to come from this sad event [30]. Finally, experience in human medicine, specifically [31], and in the cultural history of apology, generally [32], has shown that people expect a sincerely contrite individual or organization to offer to work out some form of reparation for the damages caused. At minimum, this includes seeing they are not billed for care related to the harm caused by the error.

In general, veterinary professionals and their liability insurers have not been especially concerned about malpractice complaints because of the perception that the financial risks were low. Because pets have traditionally been treated as personal property (ie, chattel) in the court system [33], the aggrieved pet owner has been entitled only to economic value (replacement cost, cost of training, costs of care, and sometimes loss of anticipated breeding revenue), even if negligence on the part of the veterinary practice can be demonstrated. Loss or damage to even a cherished item of personal property, such as a family heirloom, does not entitle an owner to sue for damages beyond the appraised value of the object. Surveys have confirmed that most pet owners view their pets as more than property, however, and, in fact, as a member of the family [13]. Legal scholars argue [2] "that [the] 'companion animals as property' syllogism used by a majority of today's courts is unacceptably arbitrary and unfair because it ignores the commonly understood reality that the relationship between human and companion animal is no more based upon economic value than is the modern parent-child relationship." Moreover, it is harder to argue that the same animal for which the veterinarian recommended $1500 worth of diagnostic and treatment care has a legal value of only $25 after its unexpected demise.

There have been a few noteworthy cases in which grieving pet owners have pursued malpractice claims seeking compensation beyond the replacement value of their animal as "property." In a few instances [20], juries recommended compensation in excess of $20,000 for the pain and suffering of the owner and recovery of veterinary expenditures. These verdicts remain quite rare. For example, courts have not allowed pet owners compensation for claims based on loss of companionship, such as might be permitted with the death of a human family member [32]. For now, it remains difficult and expensive to bring a malpractice action against a veterinarian [32]. With recoveries typically quite small, it is still difficult for a pet owner to find a plaintiff attorney interested in taking such a case on a contingent basis. That said, attorneys are taking more cases (a number of law schools are now offering courses in animal law) and presenting arguments that may appeal to judges and juries (58% of Americans own one or more pets) [4]. Because plaintiff's attorneys are the gatekeepers of the tort system, their increased availability should inevitably expand the opportunity for disgruntled pet owners to pursue their grievances. Dealing with embittered pet owners and even the threat of a malpractice action or complaint to a licensing board are enough to cause significant distress to most care providers.

In the next section, we consider the steps to take to increase the likelihood of an amicable resolution and to reduce the chances for a malpractice claim or licensing board complaint when there is a disappointing clinical outcome.

Reducing Client Disappointments Through Prevention and Early Recognition

The most effective approach to managing disappointing veterinary outcomes is through minimizing the risk for occurrence, addressing client frustrations before they escalate, and developing effective approaches for recognizing and resolving disappointments that have already occurred. Malpractice claims essentially represent an attempt by the disappointed client to seek, through legal intervention, a more equitable and satisfying resolution than he or she has achieved interacting directly with the veterinary practice.

CLIENT SATISFACTION: BASICS

The practice should ensure that it has assembled a customer service–oriented staff and veterinarians who recognize that the lifeblood of successful small animal practices is satisfied clients whose expectations are met. Superior customer service is built on a warm and welcoming demeanor by staff; a customer-friendly facility; and business and clinical procedures that are effective, understandable, and reliable, with the availability of helpful information [13].

Superior customer service includes good access for routine and acute visits and timely responses to routine and urgent telephone inquiries. This includes minimizing wait times, communicating about unexpected delays, and providing progress reports to clients about their pet's condition. Revenue-generating pet care, such as foods, grooming aids, flea control products, and identification chips, are readily accepted by clients when offered as a convenient service. A perception of opportunistic "up selling" may cast the practice as being too entrepreneurial, however, creating doubt about the necessity and advisability of diagnostic and treatment recommendations [34].

Because veterinary practice is a business, the timely and efficient collection of revenue is crucial to success. The client, however, is likely to be more familiar with the human health care encounter in which a health plan is typically intermediary, with only a copayment required at the time of service, typically for a small amount that is unrelated to the true cost of the medical service provided. As a result, discussions about costs and the collection of fees in a veterinary practice can seem mercenary unless conducted in the same warm and respectful tone expected of other veterinarian-client encounters.

BEYOND THE BASICS: SPECIFICS OF THE CLINICAL INTERACTION

Customer service basics form the underpinning of the practice's ability to manage disappointing outcomes with clients effectively. Beyond these fundamentals, the specifics of the interaction with clients and their pets in the examination room can reduce misunderstandings and disappointments or inadvertently increase their likelihood. Informed consent, client education, and shared decision making are among the most important tools for ensuring that the client is in a position to accept responsibility for choices about diagnostic and treatment plans. In the event that a disappointing medical outcome occurs or if the cost of services climbs higher than expected, the practice team needs the client to accept that he has been a partner in those decisions.

Discussions about treatment options and estimated costs should center on the perspective of the pet owner and the best interests of the patient and client [35,36]. For example, "Ms. Adams, we want to be sure that you understand the treatment options and their costs so you can make the best choices given your preferences and resources." Some practices may delegate the financial counseling tasks to a designated staff member or business office manager as is typically done in other health care settings in which insurance may not apply. For example, in orthodontic offices or laser eye surgery clinics, it is common for the clinical provider to make treatment recommendations and the designated staff member to provide the estimate and collect an initial payment and the signed agreement to proceed. Although this may work quite well in settings in which there is an established charge for a defined service, many diagnostic and treatment services in veterinary medicine are not so readily defined. Pet owners' specific preferences can be difficult to predict, and making assumptions can end in hard feelings. As a result, it is important for the veterinarian to be involved in reviewing the pros and cons of different treatment options in the practical context of the financial implications. Informed consent enables clients to make and feel responsible for choices in situations in which outcomes and ultimate costs are not always predictable.

BUILDING PARTNERSHIPS AND REDUCING DISAPPOINTMENTS: ELICITING EXPECTATIONS

Many clients arrive at the veterinarian's office with ideas about what might be going on with their pet, what health maintenance procedures they believe are valuable, and what treatment plans to expect. These ideas may be a result of previous veterinary experiences or advice, speaking with other pet owners, their own research via the Internet, or even reading or watching animal and veterinary programs on television. By eliciting the client's diagnoses, ideas, and expectations early on in the visit, the efficient veterinarian can more quickly recognize when there is likely agreement and when a diagnosis or recommendation needs further discussion so as to be accepted as reasonable.

For example, one may ask, "What were you thinking might be causing Ginger to be losing weight at this point? Was there something specific that you are expecting we would do in this visit?" The veterinarian is reaffirming the importance of taking into account the client's intuitions and expectations. Eliciting these thoughts early on cues the veterinarian to address clients' expectations more efficiently during the history taking, physical examination, and treatment planning phases of the visit.

In a similar vein, offering provisional diagnoses, the veterinarian could say, "Here's what I think is going on and why. How closely does that match what you are thinking?" If the veterinarian's assessment is different from the client's initial thoughts, "thinking aloud" during the examination cues the client to additional possibilities to consider. An example of making a diagnosis in this framework would be the following: "Ms. Johnson, now that we've had a chance to go through the history of her symptoms and do a good examination, I think it is most likely that the stomach problem has been caused by... Because we can never be 100% certain, I propose we do this for now, and I would expect that to cost no more than... We would then watch her closely over the next 2 weeks and see you again at that time if all her symptoms are not resolved. How does that sound to you?" A genuine pause to elicit the client's response is needed here to establish mutual agreement or discover if further discussion is needed. The veterinarian's responsibility is to apply science and experience to describe the treatment options and their anticipated costs and benefits. It is the client's right and responsibility to choose among the options that fit his or her preferences and circumstances.

ADDRESSING DISAPPOINTMENTS THAT HAVE ALREADY OCCURRED

In the event of a disappointing event or ultimate outcome, one of the client's questions is likely to be, "Would another veterinary practice have gone about this in the same way, with the same result?" Ironically, a client looks first to his veterinarian to evaluate the care and explain the outcome, including whether errors or other problems in the care contributed to the disappointing outcome [37]. As in human medicine, the veterinary client may now have access to multiple sources of information about animal health and veterinary medicine when trying to make sense of the disappointing outcome. This may lead to challenging questions that can provoke defensiveness in the veterinarian or staff member if the upset pet owner's need to understand what happened and why it happened is not anticipated and appreciated. Detecting disappointments as soon as possible offers the best hope for addressing them successfully. Client surveys can identify processes within the practice or specific staff behaviors that require correction. Veterinarians can ask clients for feedback about the visit before they leave: "How was your experience with us today? Is there anything that you wish we would have done differently?" Too often clients are allowed to go out the door or get off the telephone without a sense that their concern has even registered.

Defensive attempts by staff to explain away clients' complaints and to justify their own behavior may feel comforting in the moment, but such attempts ultimately lead to missed opportunities to resolve problems before they fester into lost business, negative word-of-mouth advertising, lost revenue resulting from client unwillingness to pay bills, formal complaints, and malpractice claims [38]. Resolving disagreements, disclosing and apologizing for problems in the care of the client and animal, and offering compensation or reparation when appropriate (eg, waived or reduced fees, a gift certificate for a pet store or groomer, a mediated financial settlement) can rebuild the damaged relationship and reduce the client's urge to retaliate for a perceived inequity [31].

These can be difficult conversations for a veterinarian and staff who are not intentional in their approach. When the client speaks, it is essential for the veterinarian to listen carefully and actively (ie, leaning forward with full attention, asking clarifying questions, offering short summaries to confirm or clarify understanding of the client's perspective and needs). Brief summaries can keep the veterinarian on target: "So if I understand you correctly..." A client's issue that may have been overlooked or misunderstood can then be more readily identified and corrected. We turn now to some specific examples of how this might be accomplished.

Imagine this situation. A client was told that he could come in on the way home from work to pick up his puppy, which was expected to have recovered sufficiently from being spayed earlier in the day. When the client arrives, the veterinarian does not feel comfortable in discharging the dog without evidence of adequate ability to walk and respond to its' environment. The client, in a frustrated tone of voice, tells the veterinarian that he is upset that no one called to make him aware of the change in discharge plans, adding that he left work early to arrive at the practice before closing and drove out of his way in heavy traffic. How does the thoughtful veterinarian respond in this situation?

Of course, it would have been best if staff had foreseen this problem and contacted the client early enough to head him off. Failing that, anticipating the client's reaction would allow the veterinary team to be better prepared to empathize with upset feelings and not to respond defensively. The client's upset feelings are often readily understandable if one listens carefully to the client's overall message. For example, the veterinarian could say, "I see. You remember being told this morning that because Max was the first operation of the day, he would be ready for discharge by closing time this evening. Because you've given us your work telephone number, you were expecting that we would have alerted you if there was a change and at least have saved you the frustration of a long trip over here this evening." Actively listening and then summarizing in this way accomplishes three things immediately. First, it demonstrates that the veterinarian or health care team member is committed to understanding the client's experience, reducing the client's need to repeat himself to emphasize what he feels has been minimized or missed. Second, it allows the veterinarian to manage his or her own emotions by focusing on the client's perspective and resisting the natural "fight or flight reaction" in uncomfortable or dangerous situations. Finally, it alerts the veterinarian to the aspects of the situation that are most upsetting and possibly confusing to the client and therefore needing to be addressed [39,40].

The ability and willingness to empathize with the client's view of the situation is the key to resolving the disappointment satisfactorily. Responding empathically simply means conveying that the client's perspective, concerns, frustrations, and expectations are understandable and that you wish things had gone differently now that you recognize the resulting impact on the client. Importantly, empathy does not mean or require agreement with each point that the client is making.

Here is how empathy might sound using the previous scenario: "Mr. Jones, I can understand your frustration at how this has worked out. You made the time to come all the way over here this evening, expecting to bring Max home with you only to be told that the trip was in vain. I want to say how really sorry I am that this has happened." Notice how the veterinarian's empathic response helps him or her to avoid the common trap of defensively trying to explain away all the client's frustration. For instance, imagine how Mr. Jones would have reacted to the following defensive and dismissive approach: "Well Mr. Jones, you can see that we're very busy here at the clinic, and we're just trying to do what is safe for your puppy. We can't promise how quickly a puppy will recover from anesthesia and be able to go home safely. You wouldn't want us to send your puppy home and then have a medical emergency later tonight, would you?".

Research on addressing disappointing outcomes in human medicine indicates that an expression of sympathy and, when appropriate, a frank apology are essential to resolution [41,42]. Our ethics make it clear that the client is entitled to an accurate understanding of what has happened, and to do anything else may be judged deceptive. Our most accurate understanding of what happened determines whether an empathic expression of sympathy is sufficient or whether the client is entitled to an apology that acknowledges responsibility for preventable problems with the care that contributed to the harm. When there has been no error involved, it can be useful to use such language as "I wish" to convey regret at the direction things have gone, for example, "I wish we had been able to stop the cancer with the chemotherapy as we had hoped." In the previous example of Mr. Smith, when a client is disappointed and things could have been done better, it may have been effective for the veterinarian to say, "I am really sorry that happened. I wish we had been able to reach you before you headed over here." Of course, it is much easier to listen and empathize convincingly when the veterinarian or staff member has truly opened up to the client's perspective.

Most clients' disappointments with medical outcomes do not result from negligent care. Unrealistic expectations, biologic variability, low probability risks and side effects, and the uncertainty of veterinary science are all more likely to have led to a poorer outcome than was hoped for in the care. The veterinarian's willingness to talk this through patiently and to address challenging questions calmly is key to resolving upset feelings when the care was satisfactory but the outcome was disappointing to the client.

Next, we consider what is different in the resolution of situations in which we recognize that a clear failure (business process or clinical) of the practice caused the disappointment (including an animal's injury or death). Specifically, we explore how a different kind of apology is now called for and how willingness to consider reparation may be essential to resolve these situations constructively.

WHEN ERROR HAS CAUSED HARM

We know in human medicine that physicians and health care organizations are reluctant to admit responsibility for a patient injury, even when their own investigation has indicated that preventable error is the most likely contributor [8,43,44]. News reports have suggested a similar reluctance in veterinary practice, as was publicly exposed, for example, in a *New York Times* report of a cover-up at the National Zoo [45,46]. In this instance, veterinary treatment errors had been made involving animal deaths, and medical records were subsequently altered to prevent recognition. The reluctance to disclose treatment errors often stems from feelings of guilt and shame, fear of censure and potential damage to one's reputation and business, and, especially, fear of a malpractice claim [47]. The human urge for self-preservation promotes a tendency to consider deceit as an alternative to exposing oneself to punishment.

The following is a model that we can borrow from human medicine [17] to guide clinicians and health care organizations in proactively disclosing and resolving medical and systems errors that cause harm. The acronym for the model is TEAM.

"T" stands for truth, transparency, and teamwork in approaching the problem. Truth and transparency lead to the client being given an accurate description of the harm and its causes. Teamwork involves the health care practice team working together to develop clarity about what happened and working together to follow through on all the steps necessary to resolve the matter satisfactorily with the client. For example, it can be helpful to have another staff member present with the veterinarian in what can be emotionally challenging discussions with the client. This team member can serve as support, as a witness, and even as a facilitator or mediator when necessary to keep a constructive focus throughout the discussions.

"E" stands for empathizing with the client's experiences and understanding his or her thoughts and emotions. "A" stands for making a clear apology and being accountable for problems in the care that caused harm [32]. Accountability includes describing the steps you are taking to reduce the chance of any other animal being similarly harmed. Research in human medicine affirms the importance to patients and families that something good (eg, reduction in harm to others) comes from their experience [30,48]. "M" stands for the ongoing management of the situation until the most satisfying resolution possible is reached with the client. Management may include providing ongoing clinical care or paying for it at another practice if that is the client's preference. It may include offering to work out compensation for the pet's loss. This addresses the client's sense of fairness and reduces perceptions that one has been victimized [22]. For minor harm or inconveniences, a sincere apology may be sufficient to satisfy the client that he or she has been treated in a fair manner [49].

Conversely, when a problem with the care has led to more substantial harm, working through the TEAM steps can be emotionally and practically more challenging. This may begin with the veterinarian starting the conversation with the client as follows: "Ms. Carson, we would like to explain to you what we now believe went wrong and offer our sincere apology. We also want to tell you the steps we are taking to prevent this from happening to others and see if there is more that you believe we can do to help you recover from this." When significant harm has occurred, clients appreciate the openness, the sincerity of the genuine apology, the commitment to address problems that could hurt others, and a recognition that the client is owed our help in recovering as much as possible from the harm that we are acknowledging we have caused [30,47]. In veterinary medicine, actual economic damages are typically small and many clients expect no restitution beyond relief of medical bills related to care. Depending on the form and amount of reparation that the practice and the client agree to (eg, waiver of veterinary bills versus financial compensation for losses), the practice needs to involve its liability insurance carrier. Customer service research in general [49] and health care experience in particular [30] teaches us that it is often possible to recover and actually build a stronger relationship with the client after a disappointment if the process is handled honestly, sensitively, and fairly in the customer's mind.

SUMMARY

Disappointing experiences are not uncommon in the increasingly complex setting of veterinary practice. Such variables as an increasing societal appreciation of the depth of the human-animal bond, new technologies, specialization, and the complexities and costs of care are interacting to raise expectations of what veterinary medicine can accomplish. These rising expectations call for veterinarians and health care teams with effective interaction skills to create partnerships with clients as shared decision makers. Both parties must accept the risks inherent in diagnostic and treatment decisions. Nowhere are these partnerships more tested than when disappointments occur in clinical or business processes or in unexpected medical outcomes. Managing these situations requires that health care teams be sensitive to client disappointments; accept responsibility for engaging with clients to resolve them; and act ethically, sensitively, and flexibly to reach the best resolutions possible while learning from the experience to reduce the potential for recurrence. The reward for their efforts is an enhanced capability to rebuild rapport, trust, credibility, and loyalty after disappointments and adverse outcomes. Success should translate into a more satisfying practice that builds and maintains its client base and minimizes its liability risks.

EXERCISE

To gain a better understanding of what specific practice-related actions lead to client satisfaction or disappointment, take a moment to reflect on the following questions. It is most helpful if you bring these questions to your staff meeting so that colleagues and members of the health care team can offer their perspectives to promote honest reflection and create opportunities for improvement strategies.

(1) What specific experiences do clients periodically find most frustrating or disappointing?

(2) How well do we understand the client's expectations related to the care of his or her pet during a visit or during a hospitalization?

    a. If our expectations and our clients' expectations are mismatched, what steps do we take to resolve this before beginning treatment?

(3) How do we currently share information within the practice about client frustrations so that we can see they are better resolved and not left to fester?

(4) Have we created a culture within the practice where everyone is open to feedback about their behavior and attitudes and shows willingness to correct weaknesses?

(5) When there is a disappointing or adverse clinical outcome, how forthright are we in ensuring that the client has an accurate understanding of what happened, even if this reveals problems in the care?

(6) How capable are we now of working out satisfying resolutions in situations in which a practice error has caused a pet and client harm?

    a. If there are weaknesses here, what steps do we need to build in, what flexibility do we need to develop, and what commitment do we need to reaffirm to resolve situations with adverse outcomes as well as possible with our clients?

References

[1] Zhao Y. Women soon to be majority of veterinarians. New York Times. June 9, 2002:12. Available at: http://www.anapsid.org/vets/vetdemos.html. Accessed March 11, 2006.

[2] Nunalee MMM, Weedon GR. Modern trends in veterinary malpractice: how our evolving attitudes toward non-human animals will change veterinary medicine. Animal Law 2004;10:125–61. Available at: http://www.animallaw.info/journals/jo_pdf/vol10_p125.pdf. Site accessed July 28, 2005.

[3] King LJ. It was the best of times, it was the worst of times. J Am Vet Med Assoc 2000;217(7): 302–3. Available at: http://www.ncvei.org/articlelinks/10-01-00%20NCVEI%20Updated.pdf4. Site accessed March 11, 2006.

[4] McWhinney J. The economics of pet ownership. 2006 Available at: http://www.investopedia.com/articles/pf/06/peteconomics.asp. Site accessed March 12, 2006.

[5] American Veterinary Medical Association. US pet ownership and demographics sourcebook. Schaumburg (IL): AVMA Communications Division; 2002.

[6] Ross CB, Baron-Sorensen J. Pet loss and human emotion. Philadelphia: Taylor & Francis; 1998.

[7] Beckman HB, Markakis KM, Suchman AL, et al. The doctor-patient relationships and malpractice: lessons from plaintiff depositions. Arch Intern Med 1994;154:1365–70.

[8] Gibson R, Janardan PS. The wall of silence. Washington (DC): LifeLine; 2003.

[9] Kohn L, Corrigan JM, Donaldson M, editors. To err is human: building a safer health system. Washington (DC): National Academy Press; 2000.

[10] Russell RL. Preparing veterinary students with interactive skills to effectively work with clients and staff. J Vet Med Educ 1994;21:40–3.

[11] Shaw JR, Adams CL, Bonnett BN. What can veterinarians learn from studies of physician-patient communication about veterinarian-client-patient communication? J Am Vet Med Assoc 2004;224(5):676–84.

[12] Stobbs C. Communication—key skill in practice. In Pract 2005;21:341–2.

[13] Brown JP, Silverman JD. The current and future market for veterinarians and veterinary medical services in the United States. J Am Vet Med Assoc 1999;215:161–83.

[14] Osborne CA. Client confidence in veterinarians: how can it be sustained? J Am Vet Med Assoc 2002;221(7):936–8.

[15] Messner E. What to do if you suspect vet malpractice. Washington Post. September 26, 2004. p. M03. Available at: www.washingtonpost.com/ac2/wp-dyn/A45754-2004Sep23. Accessed November 12, 2006.

[16] Brennan TA, Leape LL, et al. Incidence of adverse events and negligence in hospitalized patients: results of the Harvard medical practice study I. N Engl J Med 1991;324(6):370–6.

[17] O'Connell D, Reifsteck SW. Disclosing unexpected outcomes and medical error. J Med Pract Manage 2004;19(6):317–23.

[18] Leape L. Errors in medicine. JAMA 1994;265:1851–7.

[19] Charles SC. Coping with a medical malpractice suit. West J Med 2001;174:55–8.

[20] Wilson JF. Limited legal liability in zoonotic cases. Clinician's Brief 2005. May 2005.

[21] Parker L. When pets die at the vet, grieving owners call lawyers. USA Today. March 14, 2005. Available at: http://www.usatoday.com/news/nation/2005-03-14-pets-malpractice_x.htm.

[22] Schneider B, Bowen DE. Understanding customer delight and outrage. Sloane Management Review 1999;41(1):35–45.

[23] Huycke LI, Huycke MM. Characteristics of potential plaintiffs in malpractice litigation. Ann Intern Med 1994;120(9):792–8.

[24] Levinson W, Roter JP, Mullooly VT, et al. Physician-patient communication: the relationship with malpractice claims among primary care physicians. JAMA 1997;277(7):553–9.

[25] Hickson GB, Clayton EC, Githens PV, et al. Factors that prompted families to file claims following perinatal injury. JAMA 1992;287:1359–70.

[26] Avery JK. Lawyers tell what turns some patients litigious. Med Malpractice Rev 1985;2:35–7.

[27] Gorman C. Clients, pets and vets: communication and management. Newbury (IA): Iowa State University Press; 2000.

[28] O'Connell D, Keller V. Communication: a risk management tool. Journal of Clinical Outcomes Management 2003;6(1):35–8.

[29] Witman AB, Park DM, Hardin SB. How do patients want physicians to handle mistakes? A survey of internal medicine patients in an academic setting. Arch Intern Med 1996;156:2565–9.

[30] Vincent C, Young M, Phillips A. Why do people sue doctors: a study of patients and relatives taking legal action. Lancet 1994;343:1609–13.

[31] Kraman SS, Hamm V. Risk management: extreme honesty may be the best policy. Ann Intern Med 1999;131(12):963–7.

[32] Lazare A. On apology. Oxford (UK): Oxford University Press; 2004.

[33] Cupp RL, Dean AE. Veterinarians in the doghouse: are pet suits economically viable? The Brief 2002;31(3):6–21.

[34] Whitford RE. Future prosperity depends on consumer trust. J Am Vet Med Assoc 2004;225(12):1824–5.

[35] American Animal Hospital Association. Compliance study. Lakewood (CO): American Animal Hospital Association; 2002.

[36] Baker LH, O'Connell D, Platt FW. What else: setting the agenda for the clinical interview. Ann Intern Med 2005;143(10):766–70.

[37] Vincent C. Understanding and responding to adverse events. N Engl J Med 2003;348:1051–6.

[38] Antelyes J. Difficult clients in the next decade. J Am Vet Med Assoc 1991;198:550–2.

[39] Milani M. Practitioner-client communications: when goals conflict. California Veterinary Journal 2003;44(8):675–8.

[40] Lewis RE, Klausner JS. Non-technical competencies underlying career success as a veterinarian. J Am Vet Med Assoc 2003;222:1690–6.

[41] Robeznieks A. The power of apology. Am Med News 2003;46(28):9–10.

[42] Wojcieszac D. One med-mal resolution: simply saying "Sorry" works. 2004 Available at: www.Sorryworks.com. Accessed November 12, 2006.

[43] Lamb R, Studdert DM, Bohmer R, et al. Hospital disclosure practices: result of a national survey. Health Aff 2003;22(2):73–83.

[44] Gallagher TH, Waterman AD, Ebers AG, et al. Patients and physicians' attitudes regarding disclosure of medical errors. JAMA 2003;289(8):1001–7.

[45] Olson E. Under fire, chief will quit National Zoo. New York Times. February 26, 2004:16.

[46] Gallagher TH, Lucas M. Should we disclose harmful medical errors to patients? If so, how? Journal of Clinical Outcomes Management 2005;12(5):253–9.

[47] Colorado Physician Insurance Company. Disclosing unanticipated outcomes to patients. Copiscope 2002;11:1–3.

[48] Mazor KM, Simon SR, Yood RA, et al. Health plan members' views about the disclosure of medical errors. Ann Intern Med 2004;140:409–18.

[49] Malone M, Gwozdz J. Best practices: after the "oops"- Part 1. Press Ganey satisfaction monitor. January–February 2002. Available at: www.pressganey.com. Accessed November 12, 2006.

Vet Clin Small Anim 37 (2007) 151–164

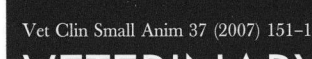

VETERINARY CLINICS
SMALL ANIMAL PRACTICE

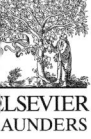

Increasing Adherence in Practice: Making Your Clients Partners in Care

Sarah K. Abood, DVM, PhD

College of Veterinary Medicine, Michigan State University, G-155 Veterinary Medical Center, East Lansing, MI 48824, USA

COMPLIANCE AND ADHERENCE: ALONG A CONTINUUM

Think about those times when you have sought medical or dental care for yourself or for a family member. Would you consider yourself a compliant patient? Do you fill and finish every prescription that is written by your physician or your dentist? Do you schedule and keep the appointment for those "benchmark" health screenings, such as twice-yearly dental cleanings, annual physical examinations, annual mammograms for women older than 40 years of age, or annual prostate checks for men 45 years of age and older? One definition of compliance is "the act of yielding to pressure" or "acquiescing to a rule, request, or demand" [1]; a more traditional use of the term *compliance* in veterinary medicine is "the consistency and accuracy with which a patient follows a prescribed regimen" [2]. The doctor-client relationship rests on the expert giving an order that the client obeys. This authoritarian relationship is at one end of a continuum of medical care (Fig. 1).

Now consider how adherent or nonadherent you are as a patient. Do you consistently brush your teeth twice each day? Do you use a membership at a gym at least once a month? Do you take a multivitamin-mineral supplement every day, or do you occasionally skip a day? Do you remember to pack supplements or medications when going on vacation? If you remember to pack them, do you remember to take them at the appropriate time while doing things out of your usual routine? Think back to the last time you filled a prescription for an antibiotic (for yourself, a family member, or a family pet); were any pills left over at the end of the prescribed time period?

Adherence is defined as the extent to which a patient continues an agreed-on mode of treatment. The World Health Organization's Adherence Project [3] recently modified this definition to include "the extent to which a person's

The author is a paid consultant to the Nestle Purina Advisory Council and received funding from Purina in 2006 for a project entitled "Dietary Recommendations: Why, When and How Are Clients Non-Adherent?"

E-mail address: aboodsar@cvm.msu.edu

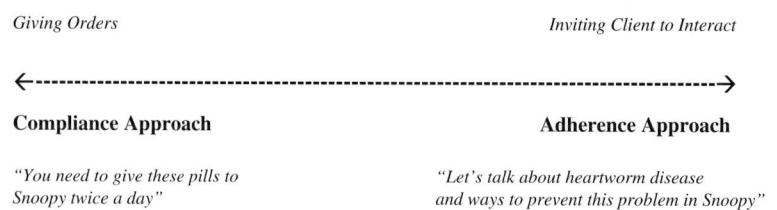

Fig. 1. Compliance and adherence along a continuum of medical care.

behavior corresponds with *agreed* recommendations from a health provider." The focus is on the relationship itself, with the doctor and client sharing and interacting and both committing to an agreed-on plan. This relationship is equal between the doctor and client and is at the other end of the continuum of medical care from compliance (see Fig. 1). The relationship-centered approach appeals to many in the health care professions because it supports their experience that patients (and clients) who are active participants in health care decision making remain committed (and adherent to) recommendations longer than those who are not.

This is not to say, however, that compliance is always "wrong" or that adherence is inherently "right." There are circumstances when compliance is essential, for example, to governmental laws and regulations (ie, rabies vaccinations) and when public safety is at risk. Few daily recommendations fall into these categories, however, leaving most to the desire and motivation of the client. This motivation depends on the quality of doctor-client interaction. Nonadherence to therapeutic recommendations is a major health care issue in human medicine; estimates of nonadherence range between 30% and 60% [4,5]. According to a review of 63 studies assessing compliance to medical interventions, close to 40% of patients took prescribed medication incorrectly or not at all and almost twice that number failed to adhere to dietary restrictions and prescribed exercise or continued to engage in compromising habits, such as smoking and abusing alcohol [6].

Few scientific studies examining client adherence have been published in the veterinary literature. Most have included small subject numbers and have evaluated client compliance to administration of short-term antimicrobials to dogs or with oral hygiene or rabies vaccination recommendations [7–12]. Defining and measuring noncompliance in scientific studies is complicated by the fact that there is no "gold standard" of measurement. Although a variety of methods have been used, problems with generating valid and reliable data remain for each of them [5,7]. Lack of patient adherence in human medicine leads to increased frustration on the part of the doctor and the patient; it also leads to incorrect diagnoses, prolonged or unnecessary treatments, increased health care costs, and decreased cost-effectiveness of interventions [6,13,14]. These same negative effects to nonadherence are considered relevant in veterinary medicine.

A recent quantitative study conducted by the American Animal Hospital Association (AAHA) found that compliance on the part of clients was much lower than what veterinarians predicted in several key areas [14]. The study examined heartworm testing, canine and feline core vaccines, preanesthetic testing, senior screenings, heartworm preventive, dental prophylaxis, and therapeutic diets. In four of the target areas, veterinarians overestimated what the actual compliance rates were in their practices. In three of the target areas, however, veterinarians underestimated owner compliance or the ability to consistently use a product in the manner it was intended (Table 1). For example, average practitioner estimates for client compliance to purchase and exclusively use therapeutic diets was 59%, but the actual overall rate was 21%; an average estimate for purchasing and using heartworm preventive was 70%, but the actual compliance rate was 48% [14]. The lack of a consistent and reliable means to measure adherence contributes to overestimating and underestimating the ability of practices to deliver the highest level of care possible. A recent publication reviewed internal practice systems and protocols that could be implemented to increase adherence to recommendations [15]. Scheduling appointments, issuing appointment reminders, receiving patients at reception and in the examination room, and conclusions for every office visit were identified as strategic "points of service," where compliance could be positively influenced by health care teams.

The differences between a compliant client and an adherent client can be subtle yet are vitally important to understanding why some animal owners do not always do what veterinarians recommend. A client may comply with the recommendation to switch an obese pet to a reduced-calorie food (he or she may, in fact, comply for months or years), but if he or she perceives that the pet does not like it, he or she may not adhere to strict feeding of that food alone. According to the AAHA study, 55% of pet owners who fed a recommended therapeutic diet supplemented that diet with other food or treats. In a more recent study, clients identified as compliant or noncompliant for purchasing a therapeutic weight loss product were surveyed in a 3.5-doctor high-volume practice in a large metropolitan area. The compliant clients were five times more likely to feed their dog or cat treats. Whether or not

Table 1
Estimated versus measured compliance rates from 2003 American Animal Hospital Association Study

Recommendation	Estimated compliance (%)	Measured compliance (%)
Heartworm testing	73	83
Core vaccines	77	87
Preanesthetic testing	66	69
Senior screenings	43	34
Heartworm prevention	70	48
Dental prophylaxis	54	35
Therapeutic diets	59	21

they were also considered adherent to all dietary recommendations is unclear, because medical records were incomplete and follow-up appointments were inconsistent or not scheduled (Kimberly Miller, personal communication, 2006).

Along the continuum of medical care from compliance to adherence, mismatches between recommendations and actions (or outcomes) are referred to as "gaps." Identifying the cause(s) of gaps between recommendations made and what the client adheres to can be valuable for recognizing opportunities to improve client interactions and the quality of patient care [15]. Challenges to adherence (or potential gaps) include economic concerns, time constraints, issues of convenience, and the ability to convince owners of the benefit of a recommendation. According to client and practitioner survey results from the 2003 AAHA study, pet owners are not the primary barrier to complying with recommendations. Although it is always true that some clients decline services because of convenience or cost, most pet owners surveyed (90%) preferred to learn about all available options first rather than just those that they could afford [14]. In contrast to some veterinarian's concerns about making multiple recommendations, only 10% of pet owners surveyed believed that recommendations were motivated by a desire to make more money [14]. Time restrictions in busy practices and misjudgments about clients' interest in providing the best possible care were two key factors associated with the failure of health care teams to make recommendations that they believed were necessary or to convince owners of the need for (and benefits of) their recommendations. Veterinary professionals could have a substantial impact on improving adherence by prioritizing and documenting the value of recommendations made and by appropriately addressing clients' concerns and questions about the recommendations made.

BENEFITS TO IMPROVING CLIENT ADHERENCE

Evidence from studies conducted over the past 30 years in human medicine clearly indicates that physicians can have a positive impact on the health-related behaviors of their patients. The core of this influence lies in effective communication skills. Effective communication between doctors and patients improves accuracy and efficiency on the part of health care providers; it also improves patient outcomes (eg, symptom relief, physiologic outcomes), increases adherence to treatment recommendations, and improves the satisfaction level of the patient and doctor with his or her interactions [16]. Although not yet widely documented, these same benefits may be realized in veterinary medicine when practitioners focus on improving communication between members of their health care team and their clients.

Enhanced adherence also improves confidence. Clients feel good about taking action and carrying out recommendations that they understand and endorse. Health care providers benefit by seeing treatment plans followed all the way to completion. Confidence on the part of the doctor, technician, and assistant further improves their ability to communicate with clients, staff, and colleagues. The veterinary practice also benefits when clients adhere to recommendations for regularly scheduled wellness and preventive care visits. It cannot be overemphasized that raising the bar for successful client adherence relies heavily on the quality of the interaction between doctors, clients, and others on the health care team.

A ROAD MAP FOR MAKING CLIENTS YOUR PARTNERS IN CARE: RELATIONSHIP BUILDING, RECOMMENDATIONS, FOLLOW-UP, AND FOLLOW-THROUGH

The four habits approach to communication skills training was established 10 years ago as a model framework for the clinical encounter in human medicine [17]. This model provides a stepwise approach to relationship building and optimizes available information for making decisions to improve patient (or client) adherence. The four habits include: (1) invest in the beginning; (2) elicit the client's perspective; (3) demonstrate empathy; and (4) invest in the end. The key goals of this approach are to build rapport and trust, efficiently exchange information, provide understanding, and increase adherence. Health care providers who develop the habit of practicing these skills during each encounter increase the likelihood of patient adherence and positive health outcomes. The four habits approach has been well documented to produce sustained improvement in patient satisfaction scores in a large health care organization [18]. It also has served as a template for validating a coding scheme to guide and measure physician communication behaviors [19]. A comprehensive review of this model, detailing the skills, techniques, and payoffs associated with each of the four habits, was recently published in the veterinary literature (Appendix 1) [20].

The first habit, invest in the beginning, focuses on engagement skills—those that establish rapport and facilitate negotiating an agenda for the visit. These skills include introductions and greetings, your style of questioning (closed- and open-ended questions), reflective listening, and identifying the client's concerns [19]. Additional skills needed to build and maintain relationships successfully include attending to body language (nonverbal cues, including yours and those of the client) and prioritizing a plan for each client visit [20].

Habit 1 Example

> Doctor: Good morning Mrs. Williams. It's nice to see you again. Let me apologize for keeping you waiting while I finished up that emergency.
> Client: Thanks. I'm in a bit of a rush this morning.
> Doctor: Yes, it seems we all are these days. How can I help you today?

The second habit, elicit the client's perspective, focuses on skills to build trust and invites clients to become active participants in the health care of their animals. These skills include assessing the client's point of view, determining reasons for seeking medical care, and exploring the impact of the animal's problem on the client's personal life [19]. Too often, veterinarians (like physicians) assume that clients (patients) are going to speak up if they do not understand or disagree with a decision. Clients (patients) want and need to be asked their opinion, and when they feel they have been heard, feelings of mutual respect occur and a partnership can develop [21].

Habit 2 Example

Client: It's LuLu Bell. She's not eating.
Doctor: Uh-huh.
Client: It's been going on for about a week and a half now.
Doctor: What do you think it could be related to?
Client: Ever since her brother, Sammy, died, she seems to have no interest in things.
Doctor: [Silence]
Client: I'm really scared that she might die of starvation.

The third habit, demonstrate empathy, focuses on continuing to build trust while allowing health care providers to be aware of their own reactions. Skills include encouraging emotional expression by the client, identifying (or naming) the client's feelings, showing good nonverbal behavior, and validating client feelings [19]. Being open to emotions and displaying verbal or nonverbal expressions of empathy can be difficult. A recent study evaluating 300 doctor-client visits revealed that only 7% of the appointments included expressions of empathy from the veterinarian [21]. Research from human medicine suggests that physicians with strong empathic skills take no more time but look for selected moments to identify and validate patient feelings [22].

Habit 3 Example

Doctor: I can understand your concern. It's frightening when a pet stops eating [empathic statement].
Client: It is. My neighbor told me he had a dog that died that way.
Doctor: I can see that you're worried, and I'll certainly talk with you more about LuLu Bell's eating. Before I do, is there anything else that you think I need to know about?
Client: No, I don't think so.

The fourth habit, invest in the end, focuses on information sharing, decision making, and following through on recommendations. Skills include giving clear explanations, using the client's frame of reference, allowing time for information to be absorbed, addressing questions, offering the rationale for tests, checking for comprehension, encouraging participation in the decision-making process, confirming the client's acceptability of the treatment plan, exploring barriers to adherence, and ending the visit with a negotiated plan for next steps [19].

Habit 4 Example

Doctor: Well, Mrs. Williams, LuLu Bell checks out fine physically, and all her laboratory work is normal. Grieving in animals is common, just as it is with us. I expect that her attitude, and her appetite, will improve within a few days. In the meantime, can you tell me what LuLu Bell's favorite foods are? Sometimes, offering some "comfort food" helps, just like it does with us.

Client: She really likes grilled chicken breast.

Doctor: That's fine for LuLu Bell. You could offer her half a grilled chicken breast with her regular food for a few days until her appetite returns and then gradually reduce it until she's eating on her own again. Does that make sense to you?

Client: Yes, it does. Thank you.

Doctor: I'll just write this recommendation down for you, and my technician, Cheryl, will call you in a couple of days to be sure things are going okay. When is the best time of day to call?

Two principal factors that influence an individual's level of readiness and commitment to adhere to a recommendation are conviction and confidence (Fig. 2). Conviction refers to one's beliefs about the value or importance of a specific recommendation. To assess client conviction, clinicians need to ask, "On a scale from 1 to 10, with 10 being of utmost importance, how valuable do you feel this special diet is to help Bruno's skin problems?" When clients demonstrate low conviction about a recommendation, they are not ready to take action. In these cases, doctors should modify goals and focus on increasing client understanding of the value of taking action. Some appropriate goals for a client with low conviction include the following:

- Ask permission to provide new information about the importance of the recommendation: "Would you be willing to hear some more information about the value of the Lyme vaccine?"
- Explore the pros and cons and the options and choices they have.
- Encourage small steps toward action.

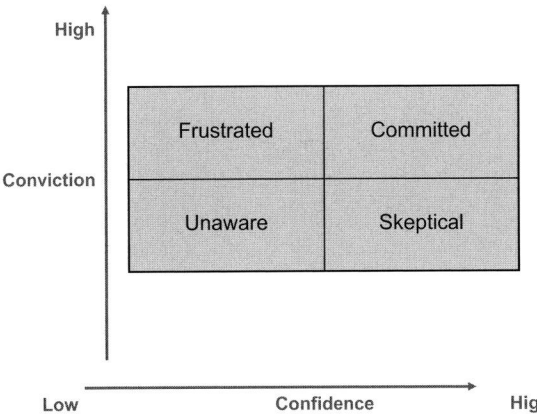

Fig. 2. Assessing client conviction and client confidence.

The second factor is confidence. Individuals have experiences that affect their level of confidence in their own ability to carry out a recommendation. For example, a client with a fear of needles is less likely to adhere to a recommendation that requires daily injections. Behavioral scientists have found that confidence is the most important determinant of successful behavior change. To assess client confidence, clinicians need to ask, "How confident are you that you can carry out this plan?"

Identifying barriers and working with the client to develop a plan to address them can be helpful. Veterinarians with limited time can defer this step to a member of the health care team with more time and expertise in problem solving. To enhance confidence, it is helpful to start with the client's own experiences by suggesting that he or she recall times when he or she has been adherent to a medical regimen for a pet (or for himself or herself). Most clients have had some level of success but tend to minimize or discount the impact of strategies previously used. Even if success was short lived, doctors can ask, "What specific things did you do that helped you?"

Enhancing communication skills through the four habits approach depends to a large extent on one's sensitivity to the client's health literacy. Health literacy is the degree to which clients are able to obtain, process, and understand basic health information well enough to make appropriate decisions (for their animals and themselves) [23]. Rates of health literacy in the United States range from 26% to 60%, and most adults aged 60 years and older have inadequate or marginal literacy skills [24–26]. Tens of millions of American adults struggle to understand basic medical terms in brochures or consent forms as well as directions on medication labels and discharge instructions [27,28]. Human patients with limited literacy skills are less likely to make use of screening tests, are more likely to present in later stages of disease, are more likely to be hospitalized, have a poorer understanding of treatment, may not be able to complete forms, and have lower adherence rates to medical regimens [28].

There are numerous "literacy sensitive" strategies that can be used by any member of the health care team [28,29]. Veterinarians and technicians who provide medical information and assistants and receptionists who may provide home care instructions can avoid assuming that every client is literate. People with limited literacy skills may compensate by trying to memorize information they have heard. If you observe a client asking for instructions to be repeated but not taking notes or not asking for written information, this may be a cue that the client has poor reading skills. Depending on one's delivery style, one or more of the following strategies may be adapted to enhance client adherence to recommendations:

- Avoid using medical jargon; use clear and simple language to describe disease conditions and treatment plans.
- Slow your delivery pace to allow clients time to process; provide information in "chunks," and "check" for understanding: "I've gone over a lot of information, and it's often hard to take it all in at once. Before I continue, I'd like to ask if you could share what you've understood so far."

- Listen and observe clients carefully for verbal and nonverbal cues: "You look like you're feeling overwhelmed by this information."
- Emphasize or demonstrate the desired behavior rather than describing medical facts: "Mix this powder with Lilly's canned food, and serve it when you eat breakfast and dinner. If you don't eat breakfast, do it right when you wake up every morning."
- When possible, provide brochures with pictures or diagrams or videotapes to show clients how to do a task at home, such as cleaning a wound site, delivering nutrition through a feeding tube, administering a pill to an animal, or cleaning ears. Finally, allow clients time to ask questions: "I'm curious what your concerns are about doing this treatment at home?"

The client's ability to recall important information, and therefore adhere to recommendations, can be improved with written instructions that make sense and are legible. Recall can also be improved if written home care instructions are duplicated for the medical record (eg, electronic medical records or carbon-copy go-home instruction forms). Instructions should be presented in the examination room rather than at the reception desk or as part of a computerized invoice. Recheck appointments should be scheduled before clients leave the hospital and included in the written home care instructions. Clients may need general information about medical or surgical conditions or specific information about home care (eg, food, water, medications, exercise—what kind, how much, and when) [30]. Prioritizing recommendations can be valuable by making clear what should clients focus on in the short term until the next visit. Guidance on when (what constitutes an emergency) and how (contact numbers or e-mail address) to contact the practice also improves adherence by providing support. Although effective written home care instructions may take some practice on the part of the doctor, they can save the practice in terms of time (minimize on time spent backtracking through medical records) and money (improve quality of care delivered, which improves results for a current medical condition) [30].

When decisions are made within a collaborative partnership, the clinician can focus on presenting the best available evidence, considering the client's perspective, and encouraging client input. Clients need to understand wellness, illness (diagnosis and prognosis), treatment options, and home care. They also need to participate in each stage of a pet's life. As clinicians, if we fail to engage or, worse, if we fail to stay connected to our clients, we risk failing the patient, the owner, ourselves, and our health care team. In contrast, engaging and staying connected with clients through the use of the four habits approach provides the best current evidence-based method for enhancing client adherence and satisfaction (Appendix 2).

Acknowledgments

The author acknowledges assistance from Dr. Tony Buffington in the preparation of this article. Background information and the figures were adapted, with permission, from veterinary educational modules developed by the Institute for Healthcare Communication (New Haven, Connecticut). Information on the

Bayer Animal Health Communication Project is available at: http://healthcarecomm.org.

APPENDIX 1. FOUR HABITS APPROACH

Habit	Skills	Techniques and Examples	Payoff
Invest in the beginning	Create rapport quickly	■ Introduce self to everyone in the room ■ Acknowledge wait ■ Convey knowledge of patient's history by commenting on prior visit or problem ■ Attend to patient's comfort ■ Make a social comment or ask a nonmedical question to put patient at ease ■ Adapt own language, pace, and posture in response to patient	■ Establishes a welcoming atmosphere ■ Allows faster access to real reason for visit ■ Increases diagnostic accuracy ■ Requires less work ■ Minimizes "Oh, by the way…" at the end of visit ■ Facilitates negotiating an agenda ■ Decreases potential for conflict
	Elicit patient's concerns	■ Start with open-ended questions: • "What would you like help with today?" Or, "I understand that you're here for … Could you tell me more about that?" • "What else?" ■ Speak directly with patient when using an interpreter	
	Plan the visit with the patient	■ Repeat concerns back to check understanding ■ Let patient know what to expect: "How about if we start with talking more about…, then I'll do an exam, and then we'll go over possible tests/ways to treat this? Sound OK?" ■ Prioritize when necessary: "Let's make sure we talk about X and Y. It sounds like you also want to make sure we cover Z. If we can't get to the other concerns, let's…"	
Elicit the patient's perspective	Ask for patient's ideas	■ Assess patient's point of view: • "What do you think is causing your symptoms?" • "What worries you most about this problem?" ■ Ask about ideas from significant others	■ Respects diversity ■ Allows patient to provide important diagnostic clues ■ Uncovers hidden concerns ■ Reveals use of alternative treatments or requests for tests ■ Improves diagnosis of depression and anxiety
	Elicit specific requests	■ Determine patient's goal in seeking care: "When you've been thinking about this visit, how were you hoping I could help?"	
	Explore the impact on the patient's life	■ Check context: "How has the illness affected your daily activities/work/family?"	
Demonstrate empathy	Be open to patient's emotions	■ Assess changes in body language and voice tone ■ Look for opportunities to use brief empathic comments or gestures	■ Adds depth and meaning to the visit ■ Builds trust, leading to better diagnostic information, adherence, and outcomes ■ Makes limit-setting or saying "no" easier
	Make at least one empathic statement	■ Name a likely emotion: "That sounds really upsetting." ■ Compliment patient on efforts to address problem	
	Convey empathy nonverbally	■ Use a pause, touch, or facial expression	
	Be aware of your own reactions	■ Use own emotional response as a clue to what patient might be feeling ■ Take a brief break if necessary	
Invest in the end	Deliver diagnostic information	■ Frame diagnosis in terms of patient's original concerns ■ Test patient's comprehension	■ Increases potential for collaboration ■ Influences health outcomes ■ Improves adherence ■ Reduces return calls and visits ■ Encourages self care
	Provide education	■ Explain rationale for tests and treatments ■ Review possible side effects and expected course of recovery ■ Recommend lifestyle changes ■ Provide written materials and refer to other sources	
	Involve patient in making decisions	■ Discuss treatment goals ■ Explore options, listening for the patient's preferences ■ Set limits respectfully: "I can understand how getting that test makes sense to you. From my point of view, since the results won't help us diagnose or treat your symptoms, I suggest we consider this instead." ■ Assess patient's ability and motivation to carry out plan	
	Complete the visit	■ Ask for additional questions: "What questions do you have?" ■ Assess satisfaction: "Did you get what you needed?" ■ Reassure patient of ongoing care	

©Physician Education & Development, TPMG, Inc. No relation to Stephen R. Covey's book, *The 7 Habits of Highly Effective People*

From Frankel RM. Pets, vets and frets: what relationship-centered care research has to offer veterinary medicine. J Vet Med Educ 2006;33(1):22; with permission.

APPENDIX 2. COMMUNICATION SKILL EXERCISE FOR IMPROVING CLIENT ADHERENCE

A practical implication for all members of the health care team is that communication skills can be taught and learned. An excellent reference for teaching and learning is the second edition of *Skills for Communicating with Patients* [16]. Many North American medical schools and some veterinary schools (eg, Michigan State University, Ontario Veterinary College, The Ohio State University) are training faculty and/or private practitioners on giving and receiving feedback for adult learners (students, interns, residents, and clinicians) who have been videotaped in standardized patient or client interviews. Some large private veterinary practices and/or specialty referral hospitals employ administrative staff with a background in human resource management; these individuals may have coaching skills on giving feedback and could be used for communication skill training too. The availability of accessible coaches for ongoing learning and reinforcement as well as tangible support from the business leadership is essential for translating experiences from the classroom into the clinical setting.

Peer observation and verbal (or written) feedback is an exercise that can provide immediate information, allowing for redirection and correction at the next patient encounter. This type of activity requires a well-defined format, including time for the peer observation report to be shared in a quiet neutral space (a private office or break room as opposed to an examination room or busy reception area). The individual being observed should identify (or describe) no more than two learning objectives to be focused on during a single observation; the observer should be focused on identifying and documenting skills associated with stated objectives so that feedback is specific and timely. Individualized feedback forms could be designed for any of the 23 skills detailed in the four habits coding scheme [19]. This coding scheme uses an uncomplicated five-point scale, with 5 representing the highest skill level. In addition to peer observation and feedback, client satisfaction surveys could be designed to assess the interpersonal interactions between your health care team and your clients.

For example, if a doctor in your practice would like to be assessed on his or her ability to explain the positive health benefits of weight loss for an obese pet and to create a mutually agreed-on plan with the client, the peer observer could use part of the four habits coding scheme to score or rate several different communication skills in a client-doctor interaction.

Habit 4: invest in the end
> Allow time to absorb: rate this individual's ability to provide the client time to process information.
> > - Score of 5: the clinician pauses after giving information, with the intent to allow the client to react and absorb it.
> > - Score of 3: the clinician pauses briefly for the client's reaction but then quickly moves on (leaving an impression that the client may not have fully absorbed the information).

- Score of 1: the clinician gives information and continues on quickly without giving the client opportunity to react (your impression is that this information is not likely to be remembered properly or fully appreciated by the client).

Give clear explanations: rate this individual's ability to provide the client with clear information on the risks of obesity and on positive health outcomes for pets that lose weight.

- Score of 5: the clinician discusses the issue of obesity and presents benefits of helping the pet to lose weight. The presentation is clear, with little or no use of jargon.
- Score of 3: the presentation contains some jargon and is somewhat difficult to understand.
- Score of 1: the information is stated in ways that are too technical or above the client's head (indicating that the client has probably not understood it fully or properly).

Involve in the client in decision making: rate this individual's ability to invite the client into the decision-making process.

- Score of 5: the clinician clearly encourages and invites the client's input into the decision-making process.
- Score of 3: the clinician shows little interest in involving the client in the decision-making process or responds to the client's attempts to be involved with relatively little enthusiasm.
- Score of 1: the clinician shows no interest in having the client's involvement or actively discourages or ignores the client's efforts to be part of decision-making process.

Explore plan acceptability: rate this individual's ability to elicit client acceptance of the plan.

- Score of 5: the clinician explores the acceptability of a weight management plan, expressing willingness to negotiate if necessary.
- Score of 3: the clinician makes a brief attempt to determine the acceptability of plan but moves on quickly.
- Score of 1: the clinician offers recommendations with little or no attempt to elicit the client's acceptance of (willingness or likelihood of following) the weight management plan.

Explores barriers: rate this individual's ability to explore barriers or problems.

- Score of 5: the clinician fully explores barriers to the implementation of a weight management plan.
- Score of 3: the clinician briefly explores barriers to the implementation of a weight management plan.
- Score of 1: the clinician does not address whether barriers exist for a weight management plan.

Plans for follow-up: rate this individual's ability to create a follow-up plan.

- Score of 5: the clinician makes clear and specific plans for a follow-up to the visit.
- Score of 3: the clinician makes references to follow-up but does not make specific plans.
- Score of 1: the clinician makes no reference to follow-up plans.

References

[1] Webster's II new riverside dictionary. Boston: Houghton Mifflin Company; 1996. p. 144.

[2] Shaw J, Boynton B. Communicating with clients: enhancing compliance. Presented at the Hill's Symposium on Dermatology. Palm Springs, California, April 2–4, 2006. Available at: www.HillsVet.com/conferenceproccedings. Accessed September 1, 2006.

[3] World Health Organization. Adherence to long-term therapies: evidence for action. Geneva (Switzerland): WHO Library Cataloguing; 2003.

[4] Roter DL, Hall JA. Doctors talking with patients/patients talking with doctors: improving communication in medical visits. Westport (CT): Auburn House; 1992.

[5] Vermeire E, Hearnshaw H, Van Royen P, et al. Patient adherence to treatment: three decades of research. A comprehensive review. J Clin Pharm Ther 2001;26:331–42.

[6] DiMatteo RM, Giordani PJ, Lepper HS, et al. Patient adherence and medical treatment outcomes: a meta-analysis. Medical Care 2002;40(9):794–811.

[7] Adams VJ, Campbell JR, Waldner CL, et al. Evaluation of client compliance with short-term administration of antimicrobials to dogs. J Am Vet Med Assoc 2005;226:567–74.

[8] Grave K, Tanem H. Compliance with short-term oral antibacterial drug treatment in dogs. J Small Anim Pract 1999;40:158–62.

[9] Nelson RS, Moshar PA, Carter ML, et al. Public awareness of rabies and compliance with pet vaccination laws in Connecticut, 1993. J Am Vet Med Assoc 1998;212:1552–5.

[10] Barter LS, Watson ADJ, Maddison JE. Owner compliance with short-term antimicrobial medication in dogs. Aust Vet J 1996a;73:227–80.

[11] Barter LS, Watson ADJ, Maddison JE. Comparison of methods to assess dog owners' therapeutic compliance. Aust Vet J 1996b;74:443–6.

[12] Miller BR, Harvey CE. Compliance with oral hygiene recommendations following periodontal treatment in client-owned dogs. J Vet Dent 1994;11:18–9.

[13] Cleemput I, Kesteloot K, DeGeest S. A review of the literature on the economics of noncompliance. Room for methodological improvement. Health Policy (New York) 2002;59:65–94.

[14] American Animal Hospital Association. The path to high-quality care. Practice tips for improving compliance. Denver (CO): American Animal Hospital Association; 2003.

[15] Wayner CJ, Heinke ML. Compliance: crafting quality care. Vet Clin Small Anim 2006;36:419–36.

[16] Silverman J, Kurtz S, Draper J. Skills for communicating with patients. 2nd edition. Abingdon (UK): Radcliffe Publishing; 2005. p. 8–9.

[17] Frankel RM, Stein TS. The four habits of highly effective clinicians: a practical guide. Kaiser Permanente Northern California Region. Oakland (CA): Physician Education and Development; 1996.

[18] Stein T, Frankel RM, Krupat E. Enhancing clinician communication skills in a large healthcare organization: a longitudinal case study. Patient Educ Couns 2005;58:4–12.

[19] Krupat E, Frankel R, Stein T, et al. The four habits coding scheme: validation of an instrument to assess clinicians' communication behavior. Patient Educ Couns 2006;62:38–45.

[20] Frankel RM. Pets, vets and frets: what relationship-centered care research has to offer veterinary medicine. J Vet Med Educ 2006;33(1):20–7.

[21] Shaw J, Adams C, Bonnett BN, et al. Use of the Roter interaction analysis system to analyze veterinary-client-patient communication in companion animal practice. J Am Vet Med Assoc 2004;225:222–9.

[22] Branch WT, Malik TK. Using 'windows of opportunities' in brief interviews to understand patients' concerns. JAMA 1993;269:1667–8.

[23] US Department of Health and Human Services. Healthy people 2010. US Department of Health and Human Services; 2000.

[24] Center for Health Care Strategies. What is health literacy? Fact sheet 2 of 9. Available at: www.chcs.org. Accessed September 8, 2006.

[25] US Department of Education. The health literacy of America's adults. Results from the 2003 national assessment of adult literacy. NCES 2006-483. 2006. Available at: www.nces. ed.gov/pubs. Accessed September 8, 2006.

[26] Baker DW, Gazmararian JA, Sudano J, et al. The association between age and health literacy among elderly persons. J Gerontol 2000;55B(Suppl):S368–74.

[27] Center for Health Care Strategies. What is health literacy? Fact sheet 4 of 9. Available at: www.chcs.org. Accessed September 8, 2006.

[28] Safeer RS, Keenan J. Health literacy: the gap between physicians and patients. Am Fam Physician 2005;72:463–8.

[29] Zagaria MAE. Low health literacy: raising awareness for optimal health communication. US Pharm 2004;10:41–8.

[30] Riegger MH. Written instructions crucial compliance step. DVM News 2005;36(1):27–30.

Vet Clin Small Anim 37 (2007) 165–179

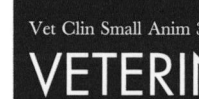

VETERINARY CLINICS
SMALL ANIMAL PRACTICE

Ethical Dilemmas in Veterinary Medicine

Carol A. Morgan, DVM[a],*, Michael McDonald, PhD[b]

[a]Interdisciplinary Studies Graduate Program, The University of British Columbia, Room 230, 6356 Agricultural Road, Vancouver, British Columbia, Canada V6T 1Z2
[b]The W. Maurice Young Centre for Applied Ethics, The University of British Columbia, 6356 Agricultural Road, Vancouver, British Columbia, Canada V6T 1Z2

E thical issues often spark emotional reactions [1,2], making communications pertaining to these issues challenging. Ethics, considered as beliefs or principles governing what is right and wrong, may be categorized according to the sphere to which they pertain: personal, social, or professional [3]. Professional ethics are set apart because professionals pledge or "profess" to uphold a societal "good" [4]. Professional status carries obligations that are "role-defined," meaning that once accepting the role of a professional, the individual promises to behave in certain ways [5]. Flowing from their professional status, veterinarians have a wide range of responsibilities, including those to clients, colleagues, the profession, and the public [3,6,7]. They also have responsibilities regarding the care and well-being of animals [8–10]. These responsibilities frequently conflict, with the result that veterinarians are constantly confronted with ethical issues. Veterinarians are "called upon to serve as an advocate of both parties' interests, even when these interests conflict" [11]. This makes veterinary ethics complex and difficult. The tension that veterinarians feel in trying to serve patients and clients has been called the fundamental question in veterinary medical ethics [3,12].

Conflicting responsibilities create what many refer to as veterinary dilemmas [11,13–20]. A moral dilemma, in a strict sense, is a conflict between responsibilities or obligations of exactly equal moral weight. In a wider sense, moral dilemmas occur when there are competing responsibilities with no obvious way to prioritize one responsibility over others. Achieving agreement about the moral weight of responsibilities to animals is difficult, because the moral status of animals is a source of profound debate [21]. Some suggest that it is nonsense to speak of moral claims for animals at all [22,23]. Others claim that animals have an important moral status in society [3,12,24]. In veterinary medicine, the moral status of animals seems to be fluid [25,26] and ambiguous [14,27,28]. This leaves interpretations of veterinarians' responsibilities open

*Corresponding author. E-mail address: camorgan@interchange.ubc.ca (C.A. Morgan).

to debate and dispute. In contrast to other professions, veterinarians must deal with a centrally contested moral claim—the moral status of animals—in their day-to-day interactions with clients and patients.

In a looser and more common sense, the term *dilemma* is used to refer to moral choices that are hard to make because of contextual factors, such as potential negative responses from clients or loss of income. These situations are not moral dilemmas in a strict sense, because an ethically correct solution is apparent but is difficult to enact. For example, a veterinarian may know that a client engages in dog fighting but chooses not to report the client to humane authorities because he or she worries that the client may retaliate by taking his or her business elsewhere or threatening extralegal action. Ethically, the obvious course of action is to report the client, because dog fighting is considered to be abuse and is illegal in most jurisdictions [3]. Beyond legal proscriptions, veterinarians are ethically responsible to reduce animal suffering [8,9]. Nevertheless, pragmatically, veterinarians worry about the actual consequences of calling humane authorities over fear of loss of income or even reprisals [29]. It is also true that these cases may be difficult to document and are often unsuccessful. Although, ethically, a clearly correct course of action exists, veterinarians may find themselves seeking other alternatives. These hard choices may also be termed *practical dilemmas*, because the right action is a difficult one to take.

In veterinary medicine, it may be difficult to separate practical and moral dilemmas. For example, some veterinarians oppose tail docking in dogs because it does not benefit the patient and causes some harm. Some of these veterinarians who oppose docking may feel compelled to perform the procedure to placate a good client, however. This is a practical dilemma. Other veterinarians view tail docking as a moral dilemma because they are uncertain how to prioritize the client's right to make decisions regarding his or her pet versus the veterinarian's responsibility to mitigate animal suffering. "Dilemmas" commonly reported in the veterinary literature are likely a combination of practical and moral dilemmas and include requests by clients to perform unnecessary procedures (cosmetic surgery), requests to perform procedures that are harmful or stressful to the animal (eg, minor surgery without anesthesia), requests for euthanasia of healthy animals, breaking client confidentiality to protect animals, and refusal by or inability of clients to provide the necessary resources (eg, financial, time, housing) for care of patients, to name only a few. Veterinarians and veterinary staff generally try to negotiate these situations with their clients in an ethically responsible and respectful way, but doing so can be challenging. Communication regarding dilemmas is an important skill for veterinarians to enable them to fulfill their professional responsibilities to patients, clients, colleagues, and the public.

SOURCES OF ETHICAL TENSION IN VETERINARY MEDICINE

When interacting with clients and staff, it is important for veterinarians to understand that there are several sources of moral dilemmas. Differences in beliefs regarding the importance of animals, differences in beliefs regarding responsibilities to animals, differences in assessment of the interests of animals, and differences in the interpretation of their professional role can all lead to ethical tension.

Differences in Valuing Animals

As already noted previously, a significant source of disagreement in veterinary medicine is the moral importance of animal well-being. Even in companion animal practice, where animals are often considered members of the family, views of the moral value or worth of animals vary from person to person. The issue is whether the interests of an animal are morally significant in their own right or only matter insofar as they are tied to the interest of human beings (eg, owners, neighbors, society). For example, some have argued that animals have no or minimally morally relevant interests because they are purely for the use of people [22,23,30]. This strongly anthropocentric (human-centered) view maintains that animals matter only insofar as they matter to people. From this perspective, companion animals may be viewed as morally significant simply because they serve the needs of people through companionship or service (therapy dogs). From an anthropocentric stance, once an animal is no longer considered useful, dispensing with the animal humanely is a morally acceptable option. Clients who claim to love their pet yet request euthanasia of a healthy animal because they are moving are likely viewing animals anthropocentrically. The pet has literally outlived its usefulness to the client.

At the opposite pole, biocentrism places significant moral value on biologic life, including animals, rather than on membership in the human species, as do anthropocentrists. These two poles create a continuum of moral inclusion ranging from humans only to all biologic life. Particularly relevant to veterinary medicine, others place significant moral weight on sentience or the ability to experience life on some conscious level [31–33]. Animals have interests in their own right quite apart from the interests of persons. The interests of food, happiness, and continued life should be counted on the same basis as similar interests in people [31,32]. Some veterinarians, veterinary staff, and clients likely have some biocentric or sentientist beliefs that animals have interests worth considering on their own merits. In general, veterinarian and client beliefs may be placed on a spectrum ranging from strongly anthropocentric views to strongly biocentric views. Clients who say "It's just a dog" and veterinarians who think "It's just a wild bird" are placing these animals in an order of moral importance. Such values underpin the degree to which people weigh the interests of animals against their own interests, for example, to save money or time. Alternatively, veterinarians may fail to offer extensive diagnostics on a hamster because they consider the animal to be less morally important (or assume that the client does) than a dog or cat. Veterinarians and clients may value animals in conflicting ways, leading to confusion or disagreement.

Differences Regarding Responsibilities to Animals

Aside from the question of the moral status of animals in relation to human beings, another source of divergence between veterinarians, staff, and clients is about the level of responsibility involved in owning or caring for an animal. Although particular individuals may agree that animals have a moral status, they may differ about human responsibilities to pets [34,35]. Most jurisdictions have legal requirements for animal care, including the provision of food, water, and shelter. How much care is owed to animals remains a source of debate, however, particularly when we move beyond the bare necessities of animal life and health. Let's assume that clients are responsible for routine preventative care (eg, immunizations, parasite control) and for treatment of at least minor injuries. Are they also responsible for treatment of complex medical problems (eg, diabetes mellitus, Cushing's disease) or for the treatment of medically complex injuries? Is the morally appropriate level of care contingent on the client's ability to pay or only on the client's willingness to pay? If the former, should clients be expected to sacrifice their interests or the interests of family members to pay for veterinary care?

Beyond defining the responsibilities that clients have to their animals, veterinarians and clients may disagree over which animals are owed these responsibilities. Many practitioners are familiar with clients who present a "stray" cat for minimal treatment only to discover that the cat has lived in the client's home for the past 10 years. It seems that some clients believe they have different responsibilities to animals that are "found" compared with those that are actively acquired. Alternatively, veterinarians may encounter clients who consent to extensive treatment of a found dog for which they plan to find a home once it recuperates, because it is "the right thing to do." Some veterinarians may discourage extensive care on the found animal because they do not believe that their client should be deemed responsible. The levels of veterinary care for which pet owners are responsible is open to debate, but so are the circumstances that activate these responsibilities.

Differences Regarding the Interests of Animals

A third source of ethical disagreement is in the assessment of an animal's "best" interests. Even when veterinarians and clients hold similar views regarding the importance of animals and responsibilities to animals, differences can occur in deciding what is best for the patient or what counts as ill health [36]. These situations parallel cases in which parents or guardians disagree with physicians regarding what counts as appropriate medical care for a child or incompetent adult (one who is not capable of making decisions because of physical or mental impairment). Clinical medical ethics focus on means and methods for determining the best outcome for a patient through substituted or proxy decision making [37]. Ethical issues include who should be making decisions and how these decisions are made [38]. Clinical ethicists work with physicians and families to articulate what may be important to the patient and in the patient's interests and whether this might be achieved through medical intervention (or not). This sort of dialogue has only just started in veterinary medicine with the recent focus of defining animal welfare and assessing quality of life in companion animals [39–43]. For example, a practitioner may firmly believe that a dog with chronic arthritis is going to benefit from long-term analgesic use; however, the owner of the dog may be more concerned with the development of side effects and refuse to medicate the animal. In this case, the veterinarian and the client both want to serve the best interests of the animal but differ on what those interests are.

Differences Regarding Veterinarian's Role

Finally, clients and veterinarians (and veterinary staff) may hold differing beliefs with respect to the ethical role that the veterinarian should play in relation to clients and patients. Some may see veterinarians as advocates for their patients, whereas others see the veterinarian as serving the client's best interests. Another view is that the veterinarian's role is merely to provide information so that clients are in a position to decide what services they want (C.A. Morgan, DVM, University of British Columbia, Vancouver, Canada, dissertation in progress) [44]. Each of these perspectives on the veterinarian's appropriate role leads to different approaches to information disclosure to clients and to the acceptability of paternalistically directing client choices. For example, a veterinarian may consider himself or herself an advocate for the patient and, based on his or her beliefs, may offer only the information likely to induce clients into making a decision that he or she believes is in the animal's best interests (C.A. Morgan, DVM, University of British Columbia, Vancouver, Canada, dissertation in progress) [44]. This veterinarian may feel perfectly justified in directing a client toward a certain treatment and decide not to disclose all available options. In the example noted previously, a practitioner may minimize or downplay potential analgesic drug side effects in treating an arthritic dog, considering that the benefits of treatment far outweigh the risks. Many clients prefer veterinarians to provide information that allows the client to make decisions, however [45]. Such clients expect the practitioner to supply information necessary for them to make a decision based on their own beliefs regarding the importance of their pet, their responsibilities to their pet, and the interests of their pet. When veterinarians, clients, and staff have conflicting notions of veterinarians' moral responsibilities, miscommunication is likely to occur.

STRATEGIES TO AVOID OR MANAGE ETHICAL TENSIONS

In medical encounters, physicians and patients communicate by using four different types of interactions, including information gathering, education and counseling, relationship building, and activation and partnership [46]. Communicating about ethical issues can involve phases similar to communications with clients about medical issues. A key step in working through ethical problems in veterinary practice is defining, or diagnosing, the source of the ethical conflict. In other words, veterinarians should attempt to gather information to discover the reason for the tension, including the commonly noted sources of tension as mentioned previously.

An essential first step in gathering information about values is to reflect on one's own beliefs, perceptions, and values [47]. Veterinarians and their staff may be unaware of their own stance regarding the standing of animals, their roles and responsibilities, and the sorts of responsibilities clients owe to their animals. Conversely, they may be under the assumption that clients (or staff) have similar views regarding animals or vice versa, leading to misinterpretations and difficulties when discussing ethical issues. Practitioners should use self-reflection to understand their own values, beliefs, and biases before engaging in this type of dialogue with clients. It may be beneficial to have these discussions during practice meetings or "decompression" sessions.

Emanuel and Emanuel [48] argue that patients in human medicine may be unaware of their own values or that these values change over time. In exploring the patient's values, a physician may be better able to provide recommendations for treatment. Further, these authors suggest that "value articulation" may include encouraging patients to consider what sort of values they ought to have rather than the values that they do have. Fulford [49] suggests that medicine should be value based as well as evidence based. Not only should the facts and scientific data count in the decision process, but the values relating to patient preferences should influence treatment plans. Just as value articulation and value-based medicine are important in the human field to ensure that human patients receive adequate support and information from their health care providers, value articulation may be even more important in veterinary medicine because of the moral fluidity and ambiguity regarding the moral status of veterinary patients. It is important for practitioners to engage clients in conversations regarding how they value their pet. For example, open-ended questions about how they obtained the animal, why they obtained the animal, and the way the animal is cared for and by whom can all provide insight into the value of the pet. It is important then to bring to the surface the beliefs and expectations of clients and, when appropriate, to explore alternative perspectives with them. Equally important is to revisit these beliefs on an ongoing basis, because values may change over time.

Once discovering the values underpinning an ethically problematic situation, practitioners may find it necessary to discuss with clients the roles and responsibilities of veterinarians. For example, clients may (mistakenly) believe that veterinarians are required to follow their wishes and directions blindly. When a veterinarian refuses to practice according to the client's wishes, for example, to extract a loose tooth without anesthesia, the client may feel confused or angry because he or she believes that the veterinarian should fulfill his or her wishes as a paying customer. That the client has an inalienable right to choose is a common perspective in veterinary practice and is bolstered by the increasing prevalence of a business orientation by practitioners. Diligent veterinarians recognize the importance of educating their clients about the responsibilities and obligations of veterinarians. In addition to the obligation to treat clients fairly, veterinarians are responsible for reducing pain and suffering in animals and for maintaining public trust by providing appropriate care to animals. Veterinarians engaging in harmful practices to animals, even at the client's request, not only adversely affect the well-being of patients but may advance the deterioration of public trust in the veterinary profession. In such situations, it is appropriate that practitioners remind clients that veterinarians have professional obligations beyond those they have to clients.

In addition to clarifying the role and responsibilities of veterinarians and veterinary staff, veterinarians may need to inform clients about responsibilities associated with pet ownership. In situations in which a veterinarian believes a client is failing to provide adequate care to an animal, the practitioner should initiate a dialogue focusing on those responsibilities. In most jurisdictions, legislation requires animal owners to provide for basic necessities. Veterinarians should be familiar with local legislation and its interpretation by the humane authorities. Beyond these bare minimums, veterinarians should consider counseling clients regarding responsibilities based on their authority as an animal health expert [50]. The type and degree of responsibilities that people have to their pets is uncharted territory in some cases, however, and veterinarians should be open to respectful dialogue with clients and not leap to conclusions.

Ideally, dialogue regarding values, roles, and responsibilities should begin early in the veterinary-client relationship. Veterinary staff may wish to find ways to demonstrate or articulate their values regarding animals, their roles and responsibilities, and expectations for clients during relationship-building phases of an appointment. Initiating this sort of dialogue before an issue arises may make moral discussion and value articulation easier in future appointments. For example, during a first meeting, a breeder of bulldogs may ask a veterinarian if he or she is willing to perform elective caesarian sections on his or her bitches. The veterinarian may take the opportunity to discuss his or her views, in an open and honest fashion, regarding management of heritable problems in purebred dogs and invite the client into the discussion. Having discussed the client's beliefs regarding animal use and responsibilities, practitioners may be able to anticipate scenarios in which ethical problems may arise. Building a rapport with clients in nonurgent circumstances may allow for better management of crises when they do occur.

The fourth task in medical encounters—activation and partnership—may serve as a useful tool in resolving difficult choices. For example, veterinarians faced with the prospect of euthanizing a healthy animal may believe that they only have two alternatives: to respect the client's wishes and agree to euthanize or to turn the client away and refuse to euthanize the pet. Because neither option actually protects the patient, some veterinarians choose the morally questionable alternative of agreeing to euthanize and then covertly find a new home for the pet. For many veterinarians, this is a significant moral dilemma. It is important for a veterinarian in this situation to explain his or her position to the client, including his or her values and beliefs about veterinarians' responsibilities for animals. He or she may then ask the client how to resolve the situation in a manner that is acceptable to all parties. Other options do exist, such as referring clients to a humane organization, assisting the client in finding a new home for the pet, or "signing" over ownership of the pet to the veterinarian. Mobilizing clients to find alternative solutions to ethical problems that have been highlighted during value articulation and responsibility clarification phases may result in win-win solutions that defuse morally problematic situations.

CREATING MORAL BOUNDARIES

Regardless of extremely effective communication surrounding ethical issues, practitioners and clients sometimes have profoundly different views regarding an acceptable course of action. At times, clients refuse all alternatives and maintain their position with respect to treatment or nontreatment. Veterinarians should feel comfortable in drawing boundaries by indicating clearly what they consider to be inappropriate solutions to a problem. There are several ways to articulate these boundaries. For example, it may be possible to develop hospital policies around issues that occur frequently, such as use of perioperative analgesia, surgery aimed at correcting behaviors (eg, debarking, declawing), cosmetic surgery, euthanasia, and questionable care (possible abuse or neglect). Common problem situations may be discussed during practice meetings to develop thoughtful and well-researched policies that all members of the veterinary team can support. It is important that veterinarians and staff understand the rationale for these policies and can articulate the reasoning to clients who seek information relevant to them.

Many ethical questions arise in nonroutine situations in which decisions are heavily context driven, such as a client's unwillingness to pursue diagnostics or treatment options. In some situations, veterinarians may believe that they cannot continue to engage in the veterinary-client relationship and may consider terminating the relationship. Doing so may have negative consequences for the patient, however. In addition, terminating the veterinarian-client-patient relationship may be impossible in some situations. For example, a client may request continued hospital care for a cat in the end stages of feline infectious peritonitis (FIP), even after repeated recommendations by the veterinarian to consider euthanasia. The client may hold religious beliefs that preclude euthanasia or may refuse to admit that his or her pet has a terminal disease. The client may even refuse to allow the veterinarian to administer analgesics or sedation to reduce the patient's suffering from fear of hastening death. In these situations, veterinarians should not accede to client requests. After clarifying their roles and responsibilities to the client and attempting to understand the client's motivation, the veterinarian may need to notify the client that failing to address pain or anxiety in a terminal condition is unacceptable. The veterinarian may need to serve the client an ultimatum that allows him or her to manage the patient's pain or, otherwise, seek outside assistance, such as humane authorities. Similarly, practitioners may encounter situations in which the level of care provided by the client is marginal and attempts to communicate with the client do not seem to have any benefit for the patient. In these cases, practitioners may need to seek the services of humane organizations while maintaining the veterinary-client patient relationship. Alternatively, a practitioner could refer his or her client to a trusted colleague in the hope that another veterinarian's opinion may influence the client rather than simply firing the client. Establishing these boundaries may highlight the importance of patient care to clients but may also minimize moral stress to practitioners.

To develop boundaries in contextually complicated situations, practitioners may apply decision-making frameworks to assist them in working through ethical issues [51–53]. These frameworks assist practitioners (and possibly clients) in working through moral questions. In larger hospitals or referral institutions, more formal mechanisms, such as ethics committees or clinical ethicists, may facilitate dialogue among veterinary staff and between veterinary staff and clients and their families [54]. Increasing the structure of ethics talk within the veterinary hospital through these more formal mechanisms may provide a level of objectivity and consistency important to increasing confidence in decisions.

SOME IMPORTANT CONSIDERATIONS

There are several important factors that veterinarians should consider when discussing ethical issues. As professionals, veterinarians hold a certain level of power in the veterinarian-client relationship not only through their knowledge and expertise but because they can limit or enable access to medications and treatments to clients and patients. It is important to remember that formal veterinary ethical and legal structures focus on ensuring the autonomy of clients and their right to make their own decisions. The informed consent doctrine requires that veterinarians provide the appropriate information to clients in a fashion that clients can understand [55]. To treat a patient well or avoid harming a patient, however, veterinarians sometimes are compelled to limit, bias, or omit information to satisfy their own needs, the veterinarian's perceived needs of the client, or the perceived needs of the patient (C.A. Morgan, DVM, University of British Columbia, Vancouver, Canada, dissertation in progress). Although limiting or biasing information may be an appealing prospect to avoid troubling situations, this "solution" reduces client autonomy and may have long-term repercussions on the veterinarian or the profession through loss of trust. For these reasons, it is important for veterinarians to discuss all morally acceptable alternatives for treatment. Some issues are subject to considerable debate within the veterinary community, and it is sometimes difficult to know whether certain alternatives are morally acceptable or not. For example, euthanasia seems to be an acceptable alternative in cases of severe illness and unacceptable in cases of mild illness. Further dialogue within the profession and between the veterinary profession and the public domain are required to clarify these areas further.

Rather than withholding or limiting information, some veterinarians may use guilt or strong persuasion to manipulate clients during ethical dilemmas. The authority that veterinarians hold as part of their professional status may allow veterinarians to significantly influence clients. Although this authority is helpful in establishing acceptable care for patients, it is possible to abuse this authority as well [50]. Veterinarians should be cognizant of this power differential when talking with clients and staff about ethical choices and avoid arbitrarily substituting their own values and beliefs for those of the clients. Although it is understandable that veterinarians may believe they have a grasp of what is "good" for an animal or the level of care that is adequate to provide for an animal, these beliefs and determinations are not the sole territory of veterinarians. Care must be taken to engender the trust of clients. If a veterinarian believes that a client may be failing in his or her responsibilities to a patient, the veterinarians should attempt to give that client frequent and fair notice of this fact. The use of assistance from outside authorities, such as the Society for the Protection of Cruelty to Animals (SPCA), should be considered a tool to benefit the situation rather than a threat or weapon.

Frequently, moral decisions involving animals are emotionally charged. Hence, it is important that veterinarians and clients recognize that the stress and anxiety surrounding veterinary visits or long workdays can affect their ability to think clearly. It is important that everyone involved has enough time to reflect on his or her own beliefs, the circumstances, and the potential alternatives to a problem. In emergency situations, this may be more difficult, but it is usually possible to mitigate patient pain, suffering, and anxiety while taking the time to make a reasoned and satisfactory decision. Hasty decisions in morally charged situations could have long-term consequences for patients, clients, veterinarians, and the profession.

SUMMARY

Veterinary medicine is rapidly evolving, and the level of care that is possible for patients is dramatically expanding. Although the perception of the importance of companion animals is changing as more people consider them family members, there is still considerable fluidity and disagreement about the moral status of animals. Practitioners and clients may disagree over the importance of animals, responsibilities owed to animals, what is best for a patient, and veterinary responsibilities. Rather than making assumptions regarding clients' beliefs or perceptions regarding any of these areas, veterinarians should become comfortable in discussing underlying values with clients (Appendix).

Because they are not professionals, clients may not understand the range of responsibilities that veterinarians hold to various parties and the importance of maintaining the public trust. Veterinarians should remind or inform clients of these responsibilities and work on building a relationship nurtured in this understanding. Being able to understand a veterinarian's dilemmas, clients may be more willing to work with the veterinarian to find solutions that work for everyone. Nonetheless, there are situations in which the communication process is unsuccessful in resolving a moral or practical dilemma. In these situations, veterinarians should be comfortable in drawing boundaries to avoid what they consider morally inappropriate action. Tools to assist veterinarians in creating boundaries include the use of practice policies, decision-making frameworks, and deferring decisions to ethics committees.

Much of this article focuses on ethical questions surrounding the treatment of veterinary patients and ways to communicate about them. These same principles may be used to manage communications around other ethical issues affecting veterinarians, including interactions with veterinary and nonveterinary staff, colleagues, and veterinary regulatory bodies. For example, a practitioner may discover that a colleague may not have the requisite skills to manage a surgical procedure. Rather than ignoring the problem or immediately contacting the regulatory authorities, the practitioner may wish to remind his or her colleague of his or her professional responsibility for competence and engage that individual in a plan to resolve the issue.

The importance of ethical issues and recognition of morally problematic situations are likely to increase as the ability to provide a high level of care escalates. As such, self-reflection on these issues by practitioners and dialogue within the profession, with clients, and within the public sphere are also likely to increase. Using the skills required for communication of medical issues is vital to elevating the dialogue of ethical issues.

APPENDIX 1
Role Play Exercise 1

As a part-time associate in a busy practice in a large urban center, your next appointment is a follow-up visit on a dog seen at the local emergency facility. In reviewing the file before the appointment, you recall meeting the patient and client the previous year. You examined the patient, a 14-year-old, male, neutered Bearded Collie cross, for otitis externa and recorded in your notes that the dog was severely matted and had extremely long nails and some fecal soiling. Your recollection of the client is an eccentric older lady who seemed oblivious to the dog's poor condition and seemed to resent your recommendation to groom him.

The dog was presented to the emergency clinic 2 weeks previously with hind limb paralysis. The emergency veterinarian's notations indicate that there "may be" a vertebral fracture and possibly discospondylitis. The dog was sent home with antibiotics, prednisone, and oral analgesics to allow the client "a little more time with him." Discharge instructions included a recommendation to recheck with the regular veterinarian in 3 days. The client chose not to bring the dog back for re-examination until 2 weeks after the emergency visit.

The client arrives at the clinic and carries the dog into the examination room on a blanket. She tells you and your receptionist that Sparky is doing well. He is eating, bright, and able to sit up. She has stopped the pain relievers because she does not believe that he is in pain. You begin to examine the dog and discover that Sparky is in lateral recumbency, he does not seem to have pain sensation in his hind limbs, he is thin and matted, and he smells like urine. Throughout the examination, the client coos to Sparky, pets him, and reassures him. You begin talking to the client by suggesting, "We need to have a conversation about quality of life." She immediately responds by saying that his life is good and that he is going to get better. After all, she "didn't kill her mother when she was elderly, and Sparky is no different." She then adds that she remembers you from the visit 6 months ago because "you didn't like Sparky because he isn't attractive." She says, aggressively, "Vets shouldn't like only the cute dogs; they should like all dogs."

Exercise

Through role play with one person acting as the client and another as the veterinarian, how would you handle the situation?

1. Identify the source of the ethical concerns.
2. Consider "diagnosing" the possible sources of ethical tension in this situation through value articulation and clarification of roles.
3. How would you resolve this situation?
4. How could this situation have been avoided?

Role Play Exercise 2

In preparation for orthopedic surgery, you open the narcotic drawer in your small suburban practice and discover that there are no narcotic patches. Because you were certain that there were at least two small patches in the drawer yesterday, you ask your technician where the patches went. Mercy, your technician, has been in your employ for 6 months and seems to be doing a great job. She breaks down and says that she used the patches on two cats that were declawed the day before because they deserved pain relief. "It's bad enough that we declaw them; we should control their pain at least," she says. You are surprised because you did not ask her to put patches on the cats. At your hospital, clients are asked to sign a consent form when they drop the cat off for surgery. The consent form has a box that clients can check if they would like to have postoperative analgesia at an additional cost of $35. The owner of the two cats that were declawed the previous day had declined narcotic patches. As this scenario unfolds, the owner of the two cats arrives to pick up her cats, both with patches still applied.

Exercise

Through role play, one person should play the veterinarian; another, the technician; and a third, the client.

What are the ethical issues in this scenario?
How should the veterinarian handle the discussion with the technician and vice versa?
What is the source of the ethical disagreement between the technician and the veterinarian?
What should the veterinarian say to the client?
How should the veterinarian respond if the client asks why postoperative anesthesia is optional?
How could this situation have been avoided?

References

[1] Haidt J. The emotional dog and its rational tail: a social intuitionist approach to moral judgment. Psychol Rev 2001;108(4):814–34.

[2] Rollin B. An introduction to veterinary ethics: theory and cases. Ames (IA): Iowa State University Press; 1999. p. 417.

[3] Koehn D. The ground of professional ethics. New York: Routledge; 1994.

[4] Wasserstrom R. Lawyers as professionals: some moral issues. In: Applebaum D, Vernon-Lawton S, editors. Ethics and the professions. Englewood Cliffs (NJ): Prentice-Hill; 1990. p. 374–84.

[5] Wilson JF. Veterinary ethics and the basics of American law. In: Nemoy JD, Fishman AJ, editors. Contracts, benefits and practice management for the veterinary profession. Yardley (PA): Priority Press; 2000. p. 1–40.

[6] Bayles MD. Professional ethics. Belmont (CA): Wadsworth; 1981.

[7] American Veterinary Medical Association. Veterinarian's oath. Schaumburg (IL): American Veterinary Medical Association; 2004.

[8] The Canadian Veterinary Medical Association. The Canadian Veterinary Oath. Available at: http://canadianveterinarians.net/about-oath.aspx. Accessed November 17, 2006.

[9] American Veterinary Medical Association. Principles of veterinary medical ethics of the American Veterinary Medical Association. Schaumburg (IL): American Veterinary Medical Association. p. 5.

[10] Tannenbaum J. Veterinary medical ethics: a focus of conflicting interests. J Soc Issues 1993;1:143–56.

[11] Rollin B. Updating veterinary ethics. J Am Vet Med Assoc 1978;173:1015–8.

[12] Tannenbaum J. Veterinary medical ethics: animal welfare, client relations, competition and collegiality. 2nd edition. St. Louis (MO): Mosby–Year Book; 1995. p. 615.

[13] Swabe J. Veterinary dilemmas: ambiguity and ambivalence in human-animal interaction. In: Podberscek AL, Paul ES, Serpell J, editors. Companion animals and us, exploring the relationships between people and pets. Cambridge (UK): Cambridge University Press; 2000. p. 292–312.

[14] Porter A. The client/patient relationship. In: Patterson D, Palmer M, editors. The status of animals: ethics, education and welfare. Wallingford (UK): CAB International; 1989. p. 174–81.

[15] Odendaal JSL. The practicing veterinarian and animal welfare as a human endeavour. Appl Anim Behav Sci 1998;59:85–91.

[16] Legood G, editor. Veterinary ethics. London: Continuum; 2000.

[17] Williams V. Conflicts of interest affecting the role of veterinarians in animal welfare. ANZCCART News 2002;15(3):1–3.

[18] Hopkins A. Ethical implications in issues and decisions in companion animal medicine. In: McCullough LB, Morris JP, editors. Implications of history and ethics to medicine—veterinary and human. Centennial Academic Assembly. College Station (TX): Texas A&M University; 1978. p. 107–14.

[19] Kingrey B. Ethical problems and decisions in food animal medicine. In: McCullough LB, Morris JP, editors. Implications of history and ethics to medicine—veterinary and human. Centennial Academic Assembly. College Station (TX): Texas A&M University; 1978. p. 115–25.

[20] Taylor A. Animals and ethics, an overview of the philosophical debate. Peterborough (Ontario, Canada): Broadview Press; 2003.

[21] Carruthers P. The animals issue: moral theory and practice. Cambridge (UK): Cambridge University Press; 1992.

[22] Narveson J. Animal rights revisited. In: Miller HB, Williams WH, editors. Ethics and animals. Clifton (NJ): Humana Press; 1983. p. 45–60.

[23] Rollin B. Animal rights and human morality. Buffalo (NY): Prometheus Books; 1992.

[24] Atwood-Harvey D. Death or declaw: dealing with moral ambiguity in a veterinary hospital. Soc Anim 2005;13(4):314–42.

[25] Sanders C. Killing with kindness: veterinary euthanasia and the social construction of personhood. Sociol Forum 1995;10(2):195–214.

[26] Heerikhuizen B, van Kruithof B, Schmidt C, et al. Dieren als een natuurlijke hulpbron: ambivalentie in de relatie tussen mens en dier, binnen en buiten de veterinaire praktijk [Animals as a natural resource: ambivalence in the human-animal relationship and veterinary practice]. In Heerikhuizen B. van Kruithof B, Schmidt C, et al., editors. Milieu als mensenwerk. Groningen (Germany): Wolters-Noordhof. (Speciale Editie Amsterdams Sociologisch Tijdschrift. 2006;23(1):12–37.)

[27] Swabe J. Animals, disease and human society: human-animal relations and the rise of veterinary medicine. New York: Routledge; 1999.

[28] Patronek GJ. Issues for veterinarians in recognizing and reporting animal neglect and abuse. In: Olson P, editor. Recognizing and reporting animal abuse: a veterinarian's guide. Englewood (NJ): American Humane Association; 1998. p. 83–100.

[29] Kant I. Lectures on ethics. New York: Harper & Row; 1963 [Infield L, Trans.].

[30] Singer P. Practical ethics. Cambridge (UK): Cambridge University Press; 1993.

[31] Singer P. Animal liberation. Singer (NY): Avon Books; 1975.

[32] Regan T. The case for animal rights. Berkeley (CA): University of California Press; 1983.

[33] Burgess-Jackson K. Doing right by our companion animals. J Ethics 1998;2:159–85.

[34] Varner G. Pets, companion animals, and domesticated partners. In: Benatar D, editor. Ethics for everyday. New York: McGraw-Hill; 2002. p. 450–75.

[35] Rollin B. The concept of illness in veterinary medicine. J Am Vet Med Assoc 1983;182: 122–5.

[36] Tonelli MR. Substituted judgments in medical practice: evidentiary standards on a sliding scale. J Law Med Ethics 1997;25:22–9.

[37] Brock DW. Good decision making for incompetent patients. Hastings Cent Rep 1994;24(6):S8–11.

[38] McMillan FD. Quality of life in animals. J Am Vet Med Assoc 2000;216(12): 1904–10.

[39] Hewson CJ. What's animal welfare science all about? Can Vet J 2004;45(3):254–8.

[40] Hewson CJ. Can we assess welfare? Can Vet J 2003;44:749–53.

[41] Hewson CJ. Focus on animal welfare. Can Vet J 2003;44(4):335–6.

[42] Wojciechowska J, Hewson CJ. Quality-of-life assessment in pet dogs. J Am Vet Med Assoc 2005;226(5):722–8.

[43] Morgan CA. Acknowledging values in veterinarian-client communications: a study in self-reports by veterinarians. Presented at the Second Annual International Conference of Communications in Veterinary Medicine. Collingwood, Ontario, Canada, July 7–10, 2005.

[44] Coe JB, Adams CL. Veterinarian-client-patient interactions: exploring the needs and expectations of veterinary clients. Presented at the Second Annual International Conference of Communications in Veterinary Medicine. Collingwood, Ontario, Canada; July 7–10, 2005.

[45] Shaw JR, Adams CL, Bonnett BN, et al. Use of the Roter interaction analysis system to analyze veterinarian-client-patient communication in companion animal practice. J Am Vet Med Assoc 2004;2:222–9.

[46] McDonald M. Medical research and ethnic minorities. Postgrad Med J 2003;70:125–6.

[47] Emanuel EJ, Emanuel LL. Four models of the physician-patient relationship. JAMA 1992;267(16):2221–6.

[48] Fulford K. Facts/values: ten principles of values-based medicine. In: Radden J, editor. The philosophy of psychiatry, a companion. New York: Oxford University Press; 2004. p. 205–34.

[49] Rollin B. The use and abuse of Aesculapian authority in veterinary medicine. J Am Vet Med Assoc 2002;220(8):1144–9.

[50] Morgan CA. A guide to moral decision making. SVME Newsletter 2006;12(1):3–4.

[51] McDonald M, Rodney P, Starzomski R. A framework for ethical decision-making: version 6.0 ethics shareware. Vancouver (British Columbia, Canada): The W. Maurice Young Centre for Applied Ethics; 2001.

[52] Rollin B. Ethics in veterinary practice. SVME Newsletter 2004;10(2):3–5.
[53] Mullen S, Main D. Principles of ethical decision-making in veterinary practice. In Pract 2001;23:394–401.
[54] Flemming DD, Scott JF. The informed consent doctrine: what veterinarians should tell their clients. J Am Vet Med Assoc 2004;9:1436–9.

Vet Clin Small Anim 37 (2007) 181–198

VETERINARY CLINICS
SMALL ANIMAL PRACTICE

Communicating with Special Populations: Children and Older Adults

Jennifer C. Brandt, MSW, LISW, PhD[a],*,
Chandra M. Grabill, PhD[b]

[a]The Ohio State University College of Veterinary Medicine, 601 Vernon Tharp Street,
Columbus, OH 43210-1089, USA
[b]Office of Academic Programs and Student Services, Michigan State University College
of Veterinary Medicine, G-155 Veterinary Medical Center, East Lansing, MI 48824, USA

V eterinary professionals must meet the growing expectations of clients to sustain success in veterinary medicine. This requires well-timed and well-delivered information about animal health care [1]. Few veterinarians, however, receive comprehensive skills training for communicating effectively with clients, particularly among special populations, such as children and the elderly. Many veterinarians believe that experience alone generates the skills necessary to discuss difficult veterinary issues, such as the serious illness, injury, or death of a pet, with pet-owning children or seniors. An increasing number of veterinary professionals have recognized a need to master requisite skills for effectively interacting with pet-owning families, however [2].

The following article on communicating with children and older adults is divided into two sections. The first section highlights the developmental benefits of the bond between children and animals and provides practical suggestions for developing child-friendly practices, including tools for helping children to cope with the death of a pet. The second section, dedicated to older adults, discusses how the developmental changes experienced by the elderly may influence encounters with veterinary professionals. The authors offer an overview of the bond between animals and seniors, issues of pet loss, and suggestions for meeting the communication needs of older adults.

CHILDREN

> From salamanders to Shetland ponies, what children learn in the company of animals exerts an enduring influence on the attitudes, values, and emotions that define us as human beings [3].

Pediatricians are not the only health care providers who encounter children in their practice. As professionals sworn to protect public health, veterinarians find

*Corresponding author. E-mail address: honoringthebond@osu.edu (J.C. Brandt).

0195-5616/07/$ – see front matter
doi:10.1016/j.cvsm.2006.09.012

that families with children represent a significant segment of the veterinary client population. A survey conducted by the American Veterinary Medical Association reported that 68.9% of households with parents and children own pets [4]. In fact, households with young couples (<45 years of age) without children were the only household type reported to have higher rates of pet ownership. Interacting with animals elicits positive benefits for children, including physical health, social and psychologic well-being, and academic achievements [5]. Children form strong attachments to pets and experience significant grief when pets die, providing important learning opportunities about life and loss [6,7].

Children are the veterinary professionals and pet caregivers of the future. Learning to communicate effectively with pet-owning parents and children can therefore be an integral component of public health education. Because pet-owning families with children vary widely in social class, cultural background, and medical literacy, targeted communication skill training is essential for veterinarians striving to interact more effectively with pet-owning parents and children.

SOCIALIZATION, EMOTIONAL DEVELOPMENT, AND NURTURANCE

Nearly 70% of US households with children own pets, and most parents report adopting an animal for the benefit of their children [8]. Kidd and Kidd [9] suggest that lifelong behaviors and attitudes toward animals evolve from these early experiences.

The Veterinarian's Oath states that veterinarians must use their "... skills for the benefit of society..." and advocates that veterinary professionals educate their clients about issues related to animal and public health [10]. Many veterinarians welcome the opportunity to discuss wellness issues directly with pet-owning parents and children. Veterinarians may be reluctant to discuss more sensitive veterinary health issues, such as chronic or terminal illness or euthanasia, in the presence of children, however.

Working in the presence of pet-owning family members, particularly children, offers many challenges to the veterinary professional. From human medicine, studies of physician interactions with parents and their ill children suggest that including children in the medical interview process promotes improved parent-child interactions as well as children's active participation and understanding in their health care [11]. It is reasonable, therefore, to suggest that educating children and their parents on important veterinary health care issues may also provide several important benefits.

For example, several studies have suggested that the use of pets in educational settings may promote the adaptive social and emotional development of children [8,12]. In a sample of 7- and 10-year-old children in California, respondents reported that they were as likely to talk to their pets about their emotions and secret experiences as with their siblings. In the same study, respondents also named, on average, two pets when asked to identify the 10 most important individuals in their lives: "...when comparing parents, friends, and pets, elementary school children considered ties with pets most likely to last 'no matter what' and 'even if you get mad at each other'" [8].

Other studies support that children in pet-owning households derive significant emotional support from their pets. For example, a sample of 10- to 14-year-old children in Michigan found that when upset, 75% of the respondents turn to their pets for support [13]. In their study of 68 5-year-old children in Indiana, Melson [8] and Melson and Schwarz [14] found that 42% spontaneously mentioned their pets when asked, "Who do you turn to when you are feeling sad, angry, happy, or wanting to share a secret?"

Animals also provide children with the opportunity to learn appropriate ways to nurture others [15]. According to parent reports, male and female children 5 to 12 years of age begin devoting decreasing amounts of time to caring for younger siblings and increasing amounts of time to pet care and play with pets [16]. Of families studied, researchers found that "...75% of 8- to 10-year-olds had sole or shared responsibility for pet care, and 92% felt that caring for their pets was an 'important' or 'very important' part of their relationship with the animal" [16,17].

DEVELOPING A CHILD-FRIENDLY BOND-CENTERED PRACTICE

Because of the significant role that the human-animal bond may play in childhood development, some veterinarians and parents are endeavoring to take an active role in helping to prepare children for a pet's visit to the "other family doctor." The veterinary team can consult specialists, such as childhood educators, counselors, or social workers, and can dedicate staff meetings or other forums to address family-centered interactions. The following suggestions may serve to facilitate this process within the practice setting [18,19]:

- Provide access to a child-oriented play area in the waiting room. Consider the use of bright colors, a playhouse or dollhouse, play materials, books, or child-sized furniture. Child- and animal-safe versions of veterinary equipment, such as a stethoscope, may also be included.
- The dress and appearance of the veterinary team can help a child to feel more comfortable in the veterinary environment. Dispensing of the white laboratory coat or wearing casual or bright-colored clothes, using a colorful stethoscope, or carrying a small stuffed animal to demonstrate or explain medical procedures can create a friendlier and less intimidating atmosphere.
- Veterinarians can develop rapport with children by asking about their favorite activities with pets, hobbies, school, or friends.
- Children aged 6 or 7 years or older may prefer a more formal approach to medical education and respond well to age-appropriate language and a reassuring tone.

PET LOSS AND CHILDREN

In a 2001 analysis of 450 calls to a pet loss and education support line, nearly 25% of callers indicated that their primary reason for contacting the hotline was to request information on how to talk with children about the illness, death, or euthanasia of a family pet [20]. Of those callers requesting information for communicating effectively with children, approximately one third were veterinarians. The remaining two thirds were parents of pet-owning children. Common questions included the following: "Should children be present for a euthanasia procedure?", "Should children be involved in the euthanasia decision-making process?", "Is it okay to lie to children about the death of their pet?", and "At what age is it appropriate to talk to children about death?" Callers indicated that the most stressful times for communicating with children about pets were at the time of diagnosis of a pet's serious or terminal illness; when pets became symptomatic and appeared "obviously sick"; and the times immediately before, during, and after a pet's death.

When a companion animal is ill or dies, parents and professionals often try to hide their emotions from children. Parents may plan to euthanize the family pet while their child is away so that when death occurs, the topic can be avoided. Instead, children may be told, "Trixie ran away." Unfortunately, when children ask for, and are denied, accurate information, they create their own answers—through imagination or information obtained from others. The longer misinformation exists, the more powerful and pervasive it becomes.

When educating parents about how to talk to their children, advise them that learning to accept illness, injury, or death is a natural experience in life. It is important that children not be "protected" from the truth or excluded from participating in family discussions of these issues. Although every child and family is different, a general understanding of how children perceive death at various ages and stages of development can be helpful in determining the appropriate timing for discussing death with children [21].

Infants and Toddlers

Infants and toddlers can and do grieve; to them, the death of someone close can be an issue of separation and abandonment [7,21,22]. They may experience sleep disturbances, regressive behavior, or volatile emotions. Parents can be encouraged to use a reassuring loving voice and gestures to show the child that someone is there to love and care for them.

Ages 3 Through 5 Years

Children aged 3 to 5 years do not understand that death is final; they know their pet is gone, but they believe it is a temporary situation. Like infants and toddlers, preschoolers need reassurance that someone is there to take care of them and that they are secure. For this age group, parents should provide simple and direct answers about a pet's death. Reading age-appropriate books to children about pet death and encouraging the expression of feelings through playing, talking, or drawing can be useful coping tools for the family as a whole.

Ages 5 Through 8 Years

Children between the ages of 5 and 8 years understand that death is final; however, they have difficulty imagining death on a personal level. At this stage of development, children may visualize death as monster or an angel. Parents can expect questions about the physical aspects of death and should not be surprised if children in this age group express anger at their pet for leaving them. Parents should be encouraged to answer questions directly. Let children know that they were loved by their pet and that it is okay to feel angry. Encourage healthy outlets for intense emotions, such as sharing favorite memories, creating a photograph album or memory book, or participating in a memorial service for their pet. Again, although every child and family is different, it may be appropriate to include children of this age group in family planning discussions about the pet. Parents can offer children an appropriate range of choices so that they can participate in the decision-making process. For example, "Ginger is sick and may die very soon. When she dies, we would like to put together a picture book that will help us to remember her. Would you like to help mommy with the picture book?"

Ages 9 Through 12 Years

Children between the ages of 9 and 12 years generally understand that death is final, personal, and something that happens to everyone. Parents can expect children in this age range to ask many questions and to have an almost "morbid" curiosity about death. Although they may seem to be coping well, preteens tend to keep many of their feelings hidden. Advise parents to provide them time and opportunities to express themselves and ask questions. Parents can encourage children of this age to gather keepsakes from their pet, write a story about their favorite memory, or keep a diary about their feelings. Encourage but do not force participation in veterinary care decision making, aftercare, and memorial service planning.

Ages 13 Through 16 Years

Because adolescents may not verbally express the intensity of their emotions, they are often mistakenly judged by their behavioral reactions to grief. Adolescents may attempt to mask their emotions from all but their closest friends. Although persons in this age group may be reticent to express their emotions, clinical studies show that teenagers often have more intense grief than any other age group [7,21,22]. Parents can help by encouraging children in this age group to participate in veterinary medical decision making and memorial service planning. Because they want to think of themselves as adults, it is important to encourage and respect their opinions and suggestions.

Decision-Making and Discussion Guidelines

Being involved in the decision-making and treatment process of a family pet that is seriously ill or injured may provide valuable lessons for children about responsibility, compassion, and commitment. Every child is unique. Thus, a variety of factors that influence the bereavement process, including age; personality; and cultural, social, and religious background, should be taken into consideration. The following are general guidelines that you can share with parents of children grieving over the death of a companion animal [7,21,22]:

- Tell children about a pet's illness, injury, or death. If children do not know why a parent or guardian is sad, they may feel at fault. Often, children worry that they are to blame: "Did I do something to make Trixie die?"
- Advise parents to answer questions honestly. Explain that every living thing can get sick or be hurt and that no living thing lasts forever.
- If a child's parents are considering euthanasia for the family pet, it is important for the parents to explain the purpose of euthanasia. Rather than saying that euthanasia is "quitting" or "stopping care," which promotes guilt and angst in children and adults, explain that euthanasia provides death with peace: "Because Tessa is suffering, we can choose to help her die with peace. It's a very sad choice to make because we love her so much, so it might help if we can think about what Tessa would want us to do for her."
- If children have questions about the euthanasia process, parents should answer them directly. For example, "Muffin is very sick and medicine won't be able to help her get better. We love Muffin very much and want to be sure that she doesn't hurt anymore. We will be taking her to the animal doctor—a veterinarian—so that he can give her medicine that helps animals to die with peace. When Muffin dies, her heart won't beat anymore; she won't be able to smell, see, walk, or feel any pain. Daddy may cry because he'll be very sad that Muffin has died. It's okay if you cry too."
- It is important for parents to avoid telling children that a pet has "gone to sleep." Because adults put children to sleep nightly, associating sleep with death creates unnecessary anxiety and may lead to disruptions in sleeping routines or behaviors.
- Avoid other euphemisms. Children are quite literal and may become confused when adults use unclear terms for death, such as "passed away," "in a better place," or "with God." Advise parents to use the "D" words, such as death and dying. They can explain that "Joey was very sick, and he died. His heart stopped beating."
- Advise parents that it is best not to schedule a pet's euthanasia procedure when the child is away from home. If this cannot be prevented for medical reasons, parents should be honest. They should avoid the temptation to say that the pet ran away from home unless this is the truth. Parents can explain that the pet was helped to die with peace and provide clear reasons for the timing of the decision.
- Generally, parents have the best sense of whether or not their child can sit still and quietly throughout the euthanasia process. Veterinarians can and should discuss their own preferences regarding a child's presence if they see that a particular child is acting out or being nonresponsive to parental requests for modified behavior. If a child is behaving in a manner that is not disruptive to the veterinary team or the euthanasia process, parents may ask the child if he or she would like to be in the room while the pet is being helped to die. Parents should let the child know that no matter what choice the child makes, his or her decision is going to be supported. Parents should be encouraged to bring an extra support person, another adult, so that if the child has a change

of heart, he or she can still be supervised appropriately while the adult family members remain with the pet.

- Know that it is alright for parents and veterinary staff to show their emotions. By discussing feelings and demonstrating honest emotions, children learn that these feelings and behaviors are acceptable. Family members should avoid ridiculing children for showing emotions or making statements that suggest children are not permitted to cry (eg, "Big boys don't cry," "Be strong for your mother").
- Let children express grief in their own way. Children may react to death with outbursts of laughter or aggressiveness or in some other manner that may be unacceptable or uncomfortable for adults. Be patient and supportive.
- It is important that parents avoid linking suffering and death with sin, punishment, and religion. Children, like adults, often feel a sense of guilt if someone dies. In addition, children have "magical thinking" and may believe that their thoughts caused the death of their pet: "If I had just [fill in the blank], Rex might still be here." Positive adult role models can help to relieve this burden of guilt by providing appropriate reassurance: "You had nothing to do with Bailey's death. He was very sick, and his lungs and heart no longer worked. At some point, all animals die."

Family-Present Euthanasia

The reality of death is visually expressed by viewing the deceased's body. Children and adults may have trouble in understanding or accepting the permanence of a pet's death unless they actually see that their pet is not "just asleep." Being present at the euthanasia procedure may also put to rest fears of what death looks like or what happens to bodies just after death. Adult role models can demonstrate to children that it is acceptable to talk with their deceased pet or to touch their pet's body. Parents and children can be encouraged to take a clipping of fur or assist with making a clay paw print as a permanent keepsake of their special companion. Offer older children the opportunity to spend some time alone with their deceased pet so that they can express their emotions privately.

More Helpful Phrases

- "Many animals don't live as long as people can."
- "It's okay you got mad at Toby for peeing on your bed. Your thoughts didn't hurt him. Toby was very sick."
- "It's okay if you made mistakes in caring for Libby. No one is perfect."
- "It's okay to laugh about your favorite memories of Cinnamon. Laughing doesn't mean that you didn't care about her."
- "How about writing a letter, telling a story, or drawing a picture of your favorite memory?"
- "How about writing a letter, telling a story, or drawing a picture of how you feel right now?"
- "It's okay to want or not to want a new pet."

Advising Families About Adopting a New Pet

Grief often feels like a ride on a roller coaster with dramatic ups and downs. It is important to advise families to proceed with caution during this phase of the grieving process. Adoption should not be considered solely as a means of diminishing the pain of loss. Taking time to talk with each family member about his or her thoughts on adopting again can send a powerful message to children that relationships are unique and irreplaceable. The time to consider adopting a new companion animal is when every member of the family has had sufficient time to deal with his or her own emotions. Adopting too soon can lead to feelings of resentment toward the new family member, who cannot take the place of the pet who has died.

OLDER ADULTS

> The bond shared with a pet can hold significant value for older adults. The pet can provide a reason for living, give social and tactile stimuli, and even function as a physical extension of the owner, operating as his eyes and ears. Pets can also be links to the past, reminding an elderly person of times shared with family and friends who are now gone [23].

Over the past century, there has been a steady increase in the proportion of the US population that is older 65 years of age, and this trend is expected to continue. In 2000, 12.5% of the population was older than 65 years of age, but by 2040, it is estimated that individuals older than 65 years of age will make up greater than 20% of the population [24]. In addition, the number of individuals who are 85 years of age or older is projected to double in size between 2002 and 2030 [24]. Although elderly individuals are less likely to own pets than are younger people [25], veterinarians are increasingly likely to work with more elderly individuals in the future because of the growing size of this age group [22]. Research in the field of human medicine has demonstrated that communication patterns between physicians and older patients are different from those with younger patients [26]. Successful veterinarians benefit from having an increased awareness of the unique needs of elderly clients that affects veterinary communication and health care [27].

Ageism, or negative attitudes about the elderly, exists throughout Western society, including medical settings [26,28,29]. In a study of ageism in human medicine, physicians were found to be less egalitarian, patient, engaged, and respectful with older clients than with younger clients [29]. Also, it has been found that human medical providers are more likely to communicate with older clients in a patronizing or condescending manner, which compromises the patient-provider relationship [30]. Veterinary professionals should be aware of their own personal biases about the elderly and attend to attitudes that can interfere with communication and veterinary care. If not, these negative messages can unintentionally cause elderly clients to feel disconnected from veterinary health professionals. In addition to attitudinal differences, generational differences in experience and knowledge can create disconnections between veterinary providers and their older clients. For example, an elderly client who grew up at a time when credit card use was not common may be surprised when credit card payment is suggested by a veterinary practice. To help "bridge" generational gaps, veterinary providers are encouraged to learn more about their clients' life experiences and appreciate the richness that can come from differences rather than assuming that the differences are problematic.

Elderly clients are likely to come to their veterinary appointments with a human companion, which creates a unique dynamic between the health care providers, the clients, and the clients' companions. In human medicine, it has been found that people older than 60 years of age are more likely than younger adults to bring companions with them to medical visits [31]. These companions often serve to provide information, help with treatment planning, and provide emotional support to clients in times of stress or strong emotion [26]. In addition, companions may dominate the interaction and detract from the clients' propensity to identify and voice their needs during health care visits. Some studies have demonstrated mixed results, including the finding that the presence of a companion reduces the amount of interaction time between physicians and elderly patients [32], whereas others have found no negative effects of the presence of companions on the doctor-patient relationship [33]. In veterinary medicine, the effect of companions has yet to be studied, although the potential for similar patterns exists. Veterinarians are encouraged to monitor their interactions with elderly clients to be sure that the clients' companions do not have a negative impact on the relationship between the veterinarians and the clients themselves. Instead, veterinary professionals can request the client's permission to enlist the companion to help to improve communication and veterinary health care delivery.

Health literacy is a term that describes the degree to which an individual can effectively understand and use health-related information [34]. Work from the field of human medicine has demonstrated that elderly individuals are more likely to have low levels of health literacy, which can have an impact on their abilities to make and follow through on important medical decisions [34]. In one study of elderly patients, as many as 34% of English-speaking adults and 54% of Spanish-speaking adults had marginal or inadequate health literacy [35]. In most cases, individuals who have low health literacy are not likely to share their deficits with their medical providers [34]. For these reasons, it is important that health providers are aware of the prevalence of low health literacy rates so that they can tailor the delivery of medical information to each client's needs. Although research on health literacy in veterinary medicine has not yet been conducted, many of the same trends could affect veterinary care. The veterinary practitioner should be alert to signs of low literacy levels of their clients and provide additional assistance to their clients when needed. Signs of low literacy include clients bringing family members with them to appointments, turning in inaccurate or incomplete forms, or claims that they have forgotten their reading glasses [34].

Although computer technology has become more prevalent in health care settings, including veterinary practices, the elderly typically have less experience with computers use than do younger clients [24]. Although the number of older Americans who have computers and Internet access is rising sharply, veterinary professionals are encouraged to ask clients about technology preferences and preferred modes of communication. For example, it would be helpful to ask clients whether they would like reminder notices to be mailed, come in the form of a telephone call, or be sent electronically via e-mail. Giving clients multiple communication options allows the provider to deliver health care messages in the manner that is most preferred by each person.

DEVELOPMENTAL ISSUES

There are numerous physical, cognitive, and social changes that occur in older adults and influence interactions with veterinary practitioners. In human medical settings, individuals who have physical, hearing, or visual deficits are more likely to be dissatisfied with their medical care than are people without these deficits [36]. Given that older adults are more likely to have age-related or disease-related deficits than are younger people, veterinarians may face unique challenges in meeting the needs of older clients [37,38].

For elderly people, typical age-related vision changes can have an impact on veterinary care. Presbyopia, or problems in visually focusing on material from a close range, is common in individuals older than 65 years of age [37,38]. As a result, older clients may have difficulty in seeing written material, which can create challenges in reading medical forms or discharge instructions. To help clients with vision problems, veterinarians may consider having large-print reference materials available for people with visual challenges. It is also important to have adequate lighting so that clients can see what is occurring during veterinary medical visits.

In addition to visual changes, hearing loss is common among the elderly. It is estimated that approximately 30% of people older than 65 year of age have some degree of hearing loss, and the prevalence of hearing problems increases with age [37]. Most elderly persons with hearing problems do not use hearing aids [39]. Older adults with hearing problems tend to have greater difficulty in hearing high-frequency sounds and confuse sounds in everyday conversation [40]. Because women's voices are generally of a higher frequency than men's voices, female health providers may have greater difficulty in being understood by elderly clients. Hearing loss can make social interactions challenging, particularly when veterinary providers are meeting with elderly individuals who may be new clients. In a study of elderly people, those who could not hear well were less satisfied with their physicians' communication than those who could hear adequately [41]. When working with the elderly, it is important for veterinary professionals to speak clearly and loudly, without yelling, so that individuals with hearing deficits are better able to comprehend. It is also helpful to make eye contact with clients so that they can read lips and pick up on nonverbal cues to enhance communication. Further, veterinary practitioners are encouraged minimize external noise in the health care setting, such as closing examination room doors and turning off overhead music, so as to reduce auditory distraction.

Older adults may also have physical changes in their mobility and may use a wheelchair or walker or may need to sit during medical examinations. When veterinary practitioners are communicating with individuals who are sitting down, it is important to consider that significant vertical height differences may inadvertently communicate a less supportive environment than is desired. These nonverbal messages become even more perceptible when difficult issues are being discussed, such as conflict, mistakes, bad news, or end-of-life issues. Rather, it is advisable for veterinary practitioners to match the vertical height of the client, which could require the veterinarian to sit or kneel to match the client's height. Veterinary practices can also create a welcoming environment for the elderly by making sure that offices and the practice materials are accessible to them. This can include having examination rooms that are accessible to individuals who are in wheelchairs. In addition, having examination tables that are adjustable can enable seated clients to see and participate in the care of their pets while the pets are undergoing examination and medical procedures [22].

It is not uncommon for older individuals to experience changes in their memory and cognitive abilities attributable to the "normal" aging process as well as to dementia [42]. To increase communication effectiveness and adherence to medical plans, veterinarians are encouraged to present information using clear and simple literacy-sensitive language and to avoid medical jargon whenever possible. The professional may find it helpful to provide large-print discharge instructions for the clients to assist in countering some of these memory deficits [22]. It is important for practitioners to work collaboratively with older clients to develop treatment plans that are easily remembered and executed. For example, if a medication needs to be given three times a day, the veterinarian can problem solve with the client about when it would be best to administer the medication. By being attentive to these challenges, veterinary communication is enhanced.

As individuals age, they are also likely to experience social and economic changes. The elderly are at risk for social isolation because of the death of significant people in their lives and the likelihood that their friends and children have moved away. Therefore, pets can play an extremely important role in the social lives of older people as a friend, a child, or a connection to other people [23]. Pet ownership itself may also create special challenges for the elderly. For example, elderly clients may need to move in with family members or to retirement and nursing care facilities that may not allow pets [23]. In doing so, elderly clients may be forced to choose between their own needs and the needs of their pets. The veterinarian is encouraged to be a resource for problem solving about housing issues and may also want to know about laws related to the presence of animals in housing complexes or nursing homes. In addition, because older adults are less likely to be working than are younger adults, they are more likely to be on "fixed" incomes. As a result, the costs of veterinary care be particularly challenging for older adults and create emotional stresses. Although veterinary professionals should still discuss all possible treatment options regardless of cost, being sensitive and respectful of the clients' choices is especially important. Effective veterinarians can help elderly clients to problem solve about ways to plan for their pet's needs through conversations about the clients' concerns, strengths, and limitations.

HUMAN-ANIMAL BOND

Over the past few decades, there has been a fair amount of research that has demonstrated the links between pet ownership and the physical, emotional, and social well-being of human beings [7,43]. There is evidence for links between pets and a variety of positive health outcomes, including decreases in cardiovascular problems, negative stress responses, and blood pressure [44]. One study found that pet owners make fewer visits to see doctors than do people who do not own pets [45]. Another study found that strong attachment to pets is negatively correlated with depression in elderly people [46]. Pets play many positive roles in the lives of elderly people [47]. In addition to companionship, pets can provide a sense of physical and emotional comfort and security for the elderly, particularly for those individuals who live alone.

Pet ownership may be a source of social contact for the elderly. The pet itself can be a source of social support, but the pet may also be a vehicle for contact with other people. In one study of elderly adults, dog owners were more likely to have more frequent social contacts compared with elderly adults who did not own dogs [48]. In this same study, older pet owners were found to have more conversations with neighbors, regardless of whether their pet was with them or not [48].

As elderly pet owners face their own changing health and housing needs, some may have concerns about how their pets are going to be cared for when they die or are unable to care for them any longer [49]. Veterinarians who work with older adults can be an excellent resource for clients to help them think through their needs. Veterinary professionals are encouraged to become informed about senior housing, assisted living facilities, and nursing homes that may allow pets. The veterinarian may also help elderly clients with these concerns to think about foster care arrangements or other short- and long-term caregiving arrangements for pets. Elderly clients who are concerned about the well-being of their pets may also want to include guardianship plans for their animals in their wills, including trusts to pay for veterinary care and food for the animals [49]. Veterinary professionals can communicate support to elderly clients through listening to clients' concerns, validating them, and providing appropriate referral resources to clients.

PET LOSS AND OLDER ADULTS

It is well known that the death of a pet can have an effect on its owner. In a survey of veterinary clients whose dogs or cats died, most clients reported that they had been affected by the death of their pet and 30% of the clients reported severe grief reactions [50]. Clients want their veterinarians to show compassion and support when their pet dies [51]. Although there have been suggestions that grief reactions to pet loss may be more severe for the elderly than for younger people, some studies have found that age is inversely correlated to level of grief [50,51]. Perhaps it is not so much the age of the owner that predicts grief reactions but the existence of other factors that influence the ways in which older people cope with pet loss. Veterinarians who are sensitive to the unique needs of elderly clients are more likely to communicate support through their words and actions [22,52].

The loss of a pet can have a significant effect on social relationships for the elderly. Research has shown that the strength of the attachment to an animal is positively correlated with the level of grief after the animal's death [50]. It has also been suggested that the elderly may have stronger attachments to their animals than do other people [53]. Elderly people who are socially isolated have more difficulty in coping with the loss than do individuals who live with other people or have adequate social support [52]. Also, for some elderly clients, the loss of their pet may represent the loss of their main social support and social contacts.

For people who are facing the anticipated or actual loss of a pet, memories and reactions to previous losses are likely to be triggered [22]. Compared with younger people, elderly individuals are likely to have encountered more losses over the course of their lifetime. Moreover, for individuals who have experienced multiple losses close in time, the loss of a pet may compound feelings of grief [23]. Given that elderly clients are likely to have owned pets in the past, they are likely to have dealt with other experiences of pet loss and euthanasia. Some of these experiences may have been handled and processed well, whereas other losses may not have been managed effectively by the owners, their support systems, or the veterinary community. When decisions about euthanasia are indicated, veterinarians are encouraged to talk with elderly clients about their previous experiences when developing treatment plans [22]. In doing so, veterinarians can ensure that clients' expectations and needs are adequately addressed.

For many elderly individuals, pet loss can also be difficult because they may not be able to take on the responsibility of another pet because of concerns about their own life span as well as economic and health issues. In many cases, elderly clients may need help in accepting the fact that they may no longer be able to own pets [7,23]. In some cases, the veterinarian may help clients to consider getting older or foster pets that may not require the long-term commitment younger pets may need.

For the elderly, the anticipated or actual death of a pet may also stir up thoughts and feelings about their own mortality. Although veterinarians may be uncomfortable with addressing these grief and loss issues, attention to these concerns can have a profound effect on clients. Veterinarians are encouraged to be aware that these are normal feelings that may come up when facing grief and loss issues with elderly clients. The veterinary professional may want to discuss the available social support for elderly clients as well as previous experiences of loss in an open way. It is also important to know that the elderly are at risk for depression and suicide, particularly in response to grief and loss [54,55]. When clients' reactions to loss are severe or prolonged or when there are concerns about suicide, referral to mental health professionals is essential.

Summary

As the number of elderly individuals in the United States increases, veterinarians are likely to have increasing opportunities to provide veterinary care to this group. Although a few individuals in the field of veterinary medicine have started to discuss the communication needs of older clients [22,27], most of the empiric work on communication has been drawn from the field of human medicine [56]. Although many of the communication strategies discussed throughout this issue are also applicable to older adults, the elderly have unique needs that can have an impact on veterinary care. Veterinary professionals with a commitment to effective client communication should have an enhanced understanding of the needs of this group.

SPECIFIC TIPS FOR WORKING WITH OLDER ADULTS

- Be aware of your own biases about the elderly, and avoid ageist language. For example, do not use condescending words that suggest the elderly are frail, childlike, and helpless.
- Be aware of possible age-related physical changes that the elderly may face.
- Be more flexible in scheduling appointments. Elderly clients may be dependent on others for transportation and may also need longer appointments.
- Help to make practices and resources accessible and welcoming to all clients (eg, offices that are easily accessible for individuals with physical disabilities, large-print resources).
- Use written materials and visual aids to complement oral communication practices. Provide simple written and visual aids for discharge materials. Follow-up with the client by means of a personal telephone call: "Please tell me what you are doing to take care of Fluffy."
- At the end of appointments, be sure to ask clients if they have any additional questions. This gives them an opportunity to raise questions or concerns that may not have come up previously. For example, "We've covered a lot if information in our appointment today. What other questions do you have about Fluffy's care?"
- When discussing euthanasia, inquire about the client's previous experiences and expectations so that you know how to meet the client's needs in the best possible manner: "Tell me about other times in your life when you've had to consider euthanizing a pet?"
- Be aware of resources in the community for elderly individuals who have to move or are concerned about long-term plans for their pets. Veterinary practices are also encouraged to have a list of referral resources that can help them to attend to the needs of older clients, including information about senior services, transportation assistance, and mental health resources.
- When a pet has died, be aware of normal grief reactions and special risks to the elderly. Make referrals to mental health professionals if necessary.

SUMMARY

Veterinarians have available to them a plethora of medical techniques, technologies, and knowledge that can help them to serve their clients and society as a whole. Among these resources, communication skills are essential for successful small animal practices. As veterinarians work with their patients, they are undoubtedly going to encounter clients in all phases of the life span. This article has focused on some of the developmental issues and factors that can have an impact on veterinary communication with children and the elderly and provides the beginning of a dialogue about possible needs of these individuals (Appendix 1). Overall, compassionate, respectful, and honest communication can enhance the relationships that veterinarians have with these important clients and advance the field of veterinary medicine.

APPENDIX 1

This exercise was adapted from customer service training games developed by Carlaw and Deming [57]. Have each member of the veterinary team walk through the practice. Instruct each individual to imagine that he or she is a young child or an elderly client. What are each member's impressions of the practice? After the walk-through, allow 10 minutes in a staff meeting for the exercise described here.

What You Need

Copy the information provided here onto an overhead or flip chart. Each participant needs a pen and paper. The facilitator needs a watch or stopwatch with the time displayed in seconds.

What To Do

Cover up all but the first question on the overhead or flip chart. You are going to reveal the questions one at a time. Remind participants to keep in mind the potential areas for change needed in the practice so as to accommodate young children and/or elderly clients better.

Advise each participant that you are going to reveal several questions or statements one at a time. Each participant should read the statement quickly and write down at least one answer. Next, quickly move to the next item on the list. The only "rule" of the exercise is to write down at least one answer to each question.

Begin the exercise by revealing the first question. Read the question to the participants, and give them the time allotted to write down a response:

1. I could serve clients with young children better if. . . [Allow 45 seconds]
2. Circle one of your answers from the previous question. [Allow 10 seconds]
3. How can you accomplish this? [Allow 45 seconds]
4. Circle one of your answers from the previous question. [Allow 10 seconds]
5. What are you willing to do to accomplish this task? [Allow 60 seconds]
6. When will you do this? [Allow 30 seconds]

Repeat this exercise by changing the first question to read, "I could serve elderly clients better if. . ."

Ask participants to read their action plans out loud, and then discuss the feasibility and timetable for implementing the plans.

Adapted from Carlaw P, Deming VK. The big book of customer service training games. New York: McGraw-Hill; 1999. p. 197–200; with permission.

References

[1] Pritchard WR, editor. Future directions for veterinary medicine. Durham (NC): Pew National Veterinary Education Program, Duke University; 1989.

[2] Bristol DG. Using alumni research to assess a veterinary curriculum and alumni employment and reward patterns. J Vet Med Educ 2002;29(1):20–7.

[3] Jalongo MR. Editorial: on behalf of children. Early Child Educ J 2004;31(4):223–5.

[4] American Veterinary Medical Association. Veterinary economic statistics. Schaumburg (IL): Center for Information Management, American Veterinary Medical Association; 1997.

[5] Jalongo MR, Astorino T, Bomboy N. Canine visitors: the influence of therapy dogs on young children's learning and well-being in classrooms and hospitals. Early Child Educ J 2004;32(1):9–16.

[6] McNicholas J, Collis GM. Children's representations of pets in their social networks. Child Care Health Dev 2001;27(3):279–94.

[7] Sharkin BS, Knox D. Pet loss: issues and implications for the psychologist. Prof Psychol Res Pr 2003;23(4):414–21.

[8] Melson GF. Child development and the human-companion animal bond. Am Behav Sci 2003;47(1):31–9.

[9] Kidd AH, Kidd RM. Developmental factors leading to positive attitudes toward wildlife and conservation. Appl Anim Behav Sci 1996;47:119–25.

[10] American Veterinary Medical Association. Available at: www.avma.org/on/news/javma/jun04/040601t.asp. Accessed July 6, 2006.

[11] Lewis C, Pantell R. Interviewing pediatric patients. In: Putnam SM, Lazare E, editors. The medical interview: clinical care, education and research. New York: Springer-Verlag; 1995. p. 209–20.

[12] Furman W. The development of children's social networks. In: Belle D, editor. Children's social networks and social supports. New York: John Wiley; 1989. p. 151–72.

[13] Covert AM, Whirren AP, Keith J, et al. Pets, early adolescents and families. Marriage Fam Rev 1985;8:95–108.

[14] Melson GF, Schwarz R. Pets as social supports for families of young children. Presented at the Annual Meeting of the Delta Society. New York, October 1994.

[15] Fogel A, Melson GF. Origins of nurturance: developmental, biological and cultural perspectives on caregiving. Hillsdale (NJ): Lawrence Erlbaum; 1986.

[16] Melson GF, Fogel A. Parental perceptions of their children's involvement with household pets. Anthrozoos 1996;9:96–106.

[17] Rost DH, Hartmann A. Children and their pets. Anthrozoos 1987;7:242–54.

[18] Lloyd M, Bor R. Communication skills for medicine. Edinburgh (UK): Churchill Livingstone; 2004.

[19] Myerscough PR. Talking with patients: a basic clinical skill. Oxford (UK): Oxford University Press; 1992.

[20] Brandt J. The Ohio State University pet loss support and information line: a summary of calls. The Hotliner Newsletter 2001;1–2.

[21] Brandt J. Helping children cope with the serious illness, injury or death of a companion animal. Columbus (OH): The Ohio State University Veterinary Teaching Hospital; 2002.

[22] Lagoni L, Butler C, Hetts S. The human animal bond and grief. Philadelphia: WB Saunders; 1994.

[23] Ross CB, Baron-Sorensen J. Pet loss and human emotion. Philadelphia: Accelerated Development; 1998.

[24] Administration on Aging, US Department of Health and Human Services. A profile of older Americans: 2005. Available at: http://www.aoa.gov/PROF/Statistics/profile/2005/2005profile.pdf. Accessed June 22, 2006.

[25] American Veterinary Medical Association. US pet ownership and demographics sourcebook. Schaumberg (IL): Membership and Field Services, American Veterinary Medical Association; 2002.

[26] Adelman RD, Greene MG, Ory MG. Communication between older patients and their physicians. Clin Geriatr Med 2000;16:1–24.

[27] Turnwald GH, Baskett JJ. Effective communication with older clients. J Am Vet Med Assoc 1996;209:725–6.

[28] Greene MG, Adelman RD. Physician-older patient communication about cancer. Patient Educ Couns 2003;50:55–60.

[29] Greene MG, Adelman R, Charon R, et al. Ageism in the medical encounter: an exploratory study of the doctor-elderly patient relationship. Lang Commun 1986;6:113–24.

[30] Ryan EB, MacLean M, Orange JB. Inappropriate accommodation in communication to elders: inferences about nonverbal correlates. Int J Aging Hum Dev 1994;39(4):273–91.

[31] Beisecker AE. Aging and the desire for information and input in medical decisions: patient consumerism in medical encounters. Gerontologist 1988;28:330–5.

[32] Beisecker AE. The influence of a companion on the doctor-elderly patient interaction. Health Commun 1989;1:55–70.

[33] Shields CG, Epstein RM, Fiscella K, et al. The influence of accompanied encounters on patient-centeredness with older patients. J Am Board Fam Pract 2005;18:344–54.

[34] Williams MV. Recognizing and overcoming inadequate health literacy, a barrier to care. Cleve Clin J Med 2002;69:415–8.

[35] Gazmararian JA, Baker DW, Williams MV, et al. Health literacy among Medicare enrollees in a managed care organization. JAMA 1999;281:545–51.

[36] Iezzoni LI, Davis RB, Soukup J, et al. Quality dimensions that most concern people with physical and sensory deficits. Arch Intern Med 2003;163(17):2085–92.

[37] Brock AM. Vision, hearing problems in the elderly. Provider 1999;25(10):101–2, 105.

[38] Raina P, Wong M, Dukeshire S, et al. Prevalence, risk factors and self-reported medical causes of seeing and hearing-related disabilities among older adults. Can J Aging 2000; 19:260–78.

[39] Bade PF. Hearing impairment and the elderly patient. Wis Med J 1991;90:516–9.

[40] Gates GA, Mills JH. Presbycusis. Lancet 2005;366:1111–20.

[41] Fook L, Morgan R, Sharma R, et al. The impact of hearing on communication. Postgrad Med J 2000;76:92–5.

[42] Park HL, O'Connell JE, Thomson RG. A systematic review of cognitive decline in the general elderly population. Int J Geriatr Psychiatry 2003;18:1121–34.

[43] Sable P. Pets, attachment, and well-being across the life cycle. Soc Work 1995;40:334–41.

[44] Friedmann E, Thomas SA, Eddy TJ. Companion animals and human health: physical and cardiovascular influences. In: Podberscek AL, Paul ES, Serpell JA, editors. Companion animals and us: exploring the relationships between people and pets. Cambridge (UK): Cambridge University Press; 2000. p. 125–42.

[45] Siegel JM. Stressful life events and use of physician services among the elderly: the moderating role of pet ownership. J Pers Soc Psychol 1990;58:1081–6.

[46] Garrity TF, Stallones L, Marx MB, et al. Pet ownership and attachment as supportive factors in the health of the elderly. Anthrozoos 1989;3(1):35–44.

[47] Enders-Slegers MJ. The meaning of companion animals: qualitative analysis of the life histories of elderly dog and cat owners. In: Podberscek AL, Paul ES, Serpell JA, editors. Companion animals and us: exploring the relationships between people and pets. Cambridge (UK): Cambridge University Press; 2000. p. 237–56.

[48] Rogers J, Hart LA, Boltz RP. The role of pet dogs in casual conversations of elderly adults. J Soc Psychol 1993;133:265–77.

[49] Greene LA, Landis J. Saying good-bye to the pet you love. Oakland (CA): New Harbinger Publications; 2003.

[50] Adams CL, Bonnett BN, Meek AH. Predictors of owner response to companion animal death in 177 clients from 14 practices in Ontario. J Am Vet Med Assoc 2000;217:1303–9.

[51] Stutts JC. Veterinarians and their human clients. J Am Vet Med Assoc 1997;210:1742–4.

[52] Quackenbush JE. Pet bereavement in older owners. In: Anderson RK, Hart BL, Hart LA, editors. The pet connection: its influence on our health and quality of life. Minneapolis (MN): Center to Study Human-Animal Relationships and Environments; 1984. p. 292–9.

[53] Carmack BJ. Pet loss and the elderly. Holist Nurs Pract 1991;5:80–7.

[54] Mulsant BH, Ganguli M. Epidemiology and diagnosis of depression in late life. J Clin Psychiatry 1999;60(Suppl 20):9–15.

[55] Bruce ML, Ten Have TR, Reynolds CF, et al. Reducing suicidal ideation and depressive symptoms in depressed older primary care patients. JAMA 2004;291:1081–91.

[56] Campbell JM, Lancaster J. Communicating effectively with older adults. Fam Community Health 1988;11(3):74–85.

[57] Carlaw P, Deming VK. Bull by the horns. In: The big book of customer service training games. New York: McGraw-Hill; 1999. p. 197–200.

Vet Clin Small Anim 37 (2007) 199–201

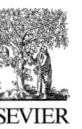

VETERINARY CLINICS
SMALL ANIMAL PRACTICE

LSEVIER
AUNDERS

INDEX

Note: Page numbers of article titles are in **boldface** type.

Moving?

Make sure your subscription moves with you!

To notify us of your new address, find your **Clinics Account Number** (located on your mailing label above your name), and contact customer service at:

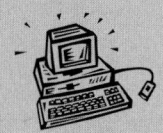

E-mail: elspcs@elsevier.com

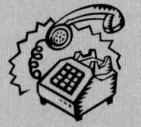

800-654-2452 (subscribers in the U.S. & Canada)
407-345-4000 (subscribers outside of the U.S. & Canada)

Fax number: 407-363-9661

Elsevier Periodicals Customer Service
6277 Sea Harbor Drive
Orlando, FL 32887-4800

*To ensure uninterrupted delivery of your subscription, please notify us at least 4 weeks in advance of move.

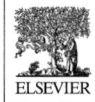
ELSEVIER